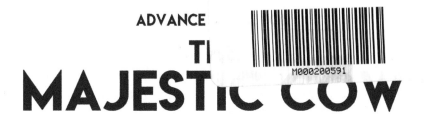

ADVANCE
THE
MAJESTIC COW

*Farmers do so much for us every day that we take for granted. It's great to see all of that hard work and our dependence on farm life get the attention it deserves in **The Majestic Cow**. See how much our lives are intertwined with farms and the hard-working folks who run them. It might change your perspective of that barn and silo you see when you drive down the highway to get something to eat.*

Brett Keisel
Pittsburgh Steeler 2002-2014
Super Bowl XL, XLIII Champion
XLV Runner Up
Beef Farmer

*Dr. Croushore's passion for telling the story of modern dairy farming is inspirational. **The Majestic Cow** is a straightforward, easy read that will open the eyes of the consuming public.*

Jonathan Lamb
Dairy Farmer and Vice President, Holstein USA

*Original, enlightening, and humorous best describes **The Majestic Cow**. Thanks to Dr. Bill Croushore for giving us an inside look at the everyday real-life experiences faced by America's farm families and veterinarians. Once you read this book you will have a new appreciation and perspective on the farm you drive by every day.*

Denny Wolff
former Pennsylvania Secretary of Agriculture
and dairy farmer.

THE
MAJESTIC COW

THE
MAJESTIC COW

A BARNYARD VET ON FARMS, FOOD, AND
THE FINEST CREATURE ON FOUR HOOVES

DR. BILL CROUSHORE

WITH JASON LILLER

Brotherton Publishing
Berlin, Pennsylvania

Published by

Brotherton Publishing
7631 Glades Pike
Berlin, PA 15530

ISBN 978-0-578-85929-3

Library of Congress Control Number: 2021932486

PHOTO CREDITS

Front cover and pages 6, 54, and 156: Jess VanGilder
Introduction: Brian Whipkey
Author photo: Suzanna Hartman, Across the Wooden
Bridge Photography

Designed and printed in the United States of America

This book is dedicated to the American farmers who, by their life's work, stamp out hunger for the American people.

And to my colleagues in the profession of veterinary medicine who, by their life's work, stamp out disease and pestilence for the American farmer.

CONTENTS

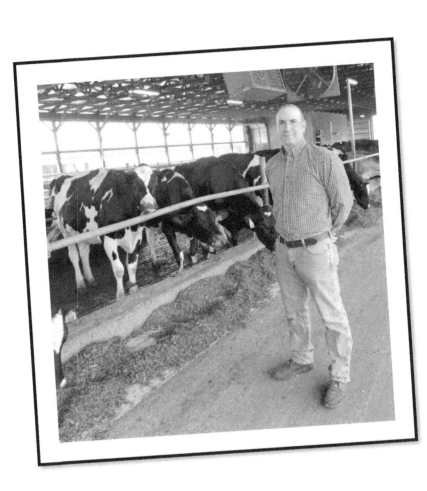

INTRODUCTION

When I tell people I'm a vet their eyes widen, they reach for my hand, and they thank me for my service.

While I sure appreciate the gratitude, I can't help but think that I'm the beneficiary of mistaken identity, so I always make sure to set the record straight: I'm the kind of vet who works with animals, a veterinarian. I don't carry a rifle. I don't wear a helmet (although sometimes I think I should). I don't take the risks or make the sacrifices that people in the military make on a regular basis in their mission to keep us safe and free. But I do have one thing in common with America's fighting forces: Like a soldier in the thick of battle, I get my boots dirty every day.

I hear what you're saying. "If you get your boots dirty every day, maybe you should sweep your exam room once in a while." I promise you that my exam room is clean and meets the highest standards for a 21st century veterinary facility. My boots get dirty because my office is the barnyard, and barnyards can get a little sloppy. I have no set hours, I have no routine, and I work until the work is done. My clients are farmers and my patients, for the most part, are cows. Now, if you're one of those people who thinks that cows are dumb, I want to make one thing perfectly clear: They are. What they lack in intelligence, they compensate with instinct. But they are also curious, affectionate, community-minded, good parents, and a friend to mankind for millennia. They provide income for farmers, a challenge for veterinarians, leather for clothing and industry, meat for everyone, and multitudes of dairy products.

Cows are also very green. Their complex digestive systems enable them to graze grass that is indigestible humans, allowing farmers to produce food without tilling up the soil. They have also been known to eat such goodies as bakery waste, distiller's grains, and spent brewery grains, things that would otherwise likely end up in a landfill.

As a species, they are incredibly diverse. Some are experts at making meat, and a lot of it. A single finished beef will yield close to five hundred pounds of meat. Other cows are experts at making milk. Pound for pound, today's dairy cow uses as much energy to produce sixty pounds of milk as a runner uses to run a marathon. The cow, however, does this every day.

Cows are bound by the chains of instinct, but that doesn't make them any less special. They are sentient, but they don't feel emotions. Nonetheless, their interactions with people are always interesting. Some are as friendly as pets; others are curious, yet cautious. Some are utterly fearful, and others are downright dangerous. The same, I guess, could be said of the human race. All things considered, you could make the argument that cows are one of the keystones of global civilization.

So I spend my days working with animals whose impact on our daily lives goes beyond what I think most people realize. As I help them through birth, diseases, disorders, accidents, and sometimes even death, I've grown to know the people who own and run the family farms that the cows call home. If you want to thank someone for their service, don't forget to thank the farmers. They have one of the most difficult, demanding jobs out there, one that requires a superhuman work ethic with no guarantee of success, little chance of steady income, no glamour, and an image that is often mocked and denigrated in the popular culture. And yet they feed a nation, year after year producing more food from less acreage and fewer workers. We have over three hundred and twenty million mouths to feed; someone has to grow the food and farmers are happy to do it.

In Pennsylvania, where I live and work, farming is woven into the fabric of daily life. We live it and breathe it (especially when the fields are being fertilized), but in many parts of the country the people don't give farming a second thought. In a way, it's nice that farming has become so efficient and productive that it can operate in the background without us having to wonder where our next meal will come from. But when we lack a basic understanding of how farms operate, we make ourselves susceptible to manipulation by anyone who has an agenda and a platform, and that's a lot of people. The stated goal of the animal-rights movement is to end meat consumption, plain and simple. Anti-GMO advocates seek to outlaw the technologies that allow farmers to grow more food on less land, thereby staving off hunger for millions of people while preserving countless acres of wilderness. The more we know about farming, the more intelligently we can consider the arguments and objections that are thrown at us in the mass media, internet, and social media every day.

A century ago, we were an agrarian society. Migration to the city in the quest for prosperity left just a small percentage of us with the responsibility of farming. Most estimates put that number at between one and two percent of our citizens. In fact, most Americans are several generations removed from the farm, but it's likely that at least your grandparent or great-grandparent was a farmer.

It's time for all of us to get back to the farm, even if only for a little bit, and even if it's only through the pages of a book. Because I have the privilege of being a veterinarian, I have learned to love and respect cows; and through my work with cows, I have learned to love and respect the family farm and the hardworking people who run it. I think you will, too. So hop in the pickup. I cleared off the passenger seat. It's a nice day; feel free to roll down the window. The fields are green, the air is clear, and there's a sweet breeze. The farm is just around the corner. Turn the page and we'll be there.

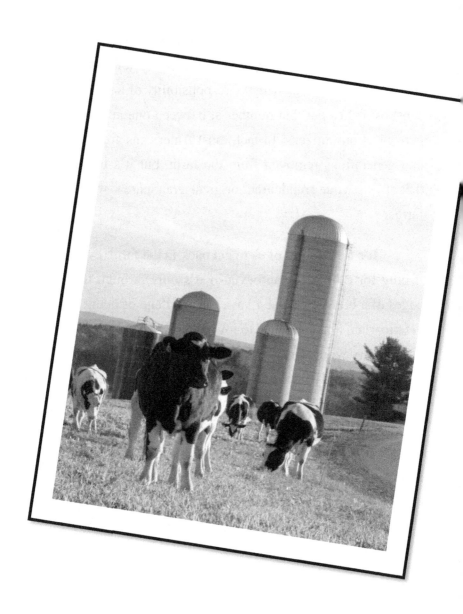

Part One

DOWN ON THE FARM

The family farm holds a special place in the hearts of Americans. It's Norman Rockwell and Grandma Moses, it's *Green Acres* and Dorothy's home in *The Wizard of Oz*, it's "The Farmer in the Dell" and "Old MacDonald." It's the root of all that's good and right with America. And yet, every year, fewer and fewer of us have a personal connection to it. The days when the US was a largely agrarian society are now far behind us. The proportion of our population that owns or works on a family farm is tiny; in some places it's hard to find a person who even has a second-hand connection to farming. We've become so urbanized and industrialized that our population at large has lost connection with where their food comes from. But the farms are still there, they're still feeding a hungry nation, and I have a front-row seat.

From the road, most American family farms still have that charming, pastoral quality, but get a little closer and you'll see that they're beehives of activity, with lots of moving parts and a whole cast of characters who keep them running. While the actual job of farming is done by only about one percent of our population nationally, support and service for farming is provided by many more people. Just in my area of Pennsylvania, there are hoof trimmers, artificial inseminators, nutritionists, custom heifer growers, and custom croppers among others.

Professional hoof trimmers periodically trim the hooves of most dairy and some beef cattle to maintain proper hoof conformation. They also treat any infections they might find during the process. Artificial inseminators have the task of breeding the cows and heifers when they are in heat in the case where a farmer doesn't keep a bull on the farm. Nutritionists sample forages and develop the proper ration for the cows and heifers. Custom heifer growers raise the young stock to free up time for the farm's dairy operation. Custom croppers provide planting and harvesting services to produce the feed for livestock farmers who may not have the time or the equipment for the job.

And it doesn't end there. There are also milk haulers, milk testers, milk inspectors, cow milkers, (*somebody* has to milk them), milk processors, and milking equipment servicepeople.

The list goes on. There are herdsmen, seed salespeople, fertilizer dealers, pesticide applicators, pharmaceutical representatives, crop specialists, and agronomists. Consultants, extension agents, veterinarians, accountants, and bankers provide technical expertise, information, and hopefully wisdom to their clients, the farmers. Equipment dealers, barn service technicians, manure haulers, hay dealers, and feed mill workers are also essential cogs in the wheel that grows our food.

The variety of farmers is nearly as extensive as their supporting cast. There are dairy farmers, beef farmers, poultry farmers, hog farmers, goat farmers, sheep herders, and llama and alpaca breeders. There are also trout, catfish, crayfish, and other fish farmers. We have grain farmers, produce farmers, potato farmers, and flower farmers. Apples, pears, peaches, plums, citrus fruits, and nuts have to be farmed too. And, of course, if there are animals on the farm, the veterinarian is essential. But as essential as I am, I am still just one small part of a great big machine, one that's been running for a long, long time.

Indeed, only about one percent of the American population are farmers and the supporting cast is not much larger. The optimist in me says that, even though most people are two or three generations removed from the farm, they are still *only* two or three generations removed. I smell opportunity there as the farm is still an object of curiosity, even if it is misunderstood at times.

One of the most striking misunderstandings of agriculture is that of the "factory farm." In our country, 98% of farms are still family owned, yet there is the perception that our food is grown on corporate factories. The pejorative term "factory farm" implies anything but pastoral. But what is a factory farm?

Maybe it's size that constitutes a factory farm. At what size does a farm becomes a factory? Unless there is evidence to the contrary, that determination is arbitrary. The average dairy herd in Pennsylvania today is about eighty cows, depending on the source. By contrast, the average herd size in Pennsylvania forty years ago was about twenty-three cows. Was an eighty-cow dairy considered a factory a mere forty years ago? Or maybe automation characterizes a farm as a factory. But most farms I visit have some degree of automation employed to reduce toil. Does the presence of hired workers make a farm a factory? If so, very few farms exist today without the benefit of hired labor, even if it's a high school kid to help bale hay or feed the calves. Factory farms surely make use of the latest technologies, but so does every farm on which I step foot.

My point is that the term "factory farm" is a derogatory term intended to paint an ambiguous picture of steel buildings, smokestacks and machines churning out processed burgers and nuggets. There's nothing pastoral about a factory, but that's not what farms are.

Folks who are two or three generations removed from the farm still recall the pastoral setting and it surely brings back fond memories of family gatherings, good food and a slower pace. Those are wonderful things, but that isn't agriculture today. Nor could it be for reasons we will see.

WHEN WAS THE GOLDEN AGE OF FARMING?

If there was a golden age of farming, when would it have been? Would it be when people first learned to plant and cultivate grains resulting in the growth of civilization? Or maybe it would be when the internal combustion engine replaced teams of draft horses? Or was it when technology took over as the driving force behind production, lifting it to heights that were unimaginable just a generation before?

I really don't know the answer; that's why I posed the question. Farming began as a means to reduce toil, the toil associated with the hunting and gathering of food. Its result was the opportunity for some people to pursue other endeavors, like inventing wheels and kindling fires. Well, maybe those came about even before farming, but you get my drift. Regardless of what you may have heard, farming is the oldest profession.

But tilling the ground by hand and sowing seeds without the benefit of tools was not easy. You might even say it was toil. So, in the never-ending quest to reduce toil, farmers enlisted the help of horses for draft and the aid of tools to work the ground. Yields increased. This could be the golden age.

Still, it was difficult. Horses required training and they could only do so much. The tools were rudimentary and inefficient. Yields probably didn't increase much over the centuries and people were still susceptible to famine and starvation. Storage options were limited and there wasn't much variety in the food supply.

Then came the industrial revolution. Maybe *this* was the golden age of agriculture. Farmers could get twice as much done with half as much work as before. Yields increased again.

The breakthroughs kept coming. In the early twentieth century, two chemists discovered the process of making nitrogen fertilizer from the nitrogen in the air. It is called the Haber-Bosch process and resulted in the Green Revolution. Farmers could now purchase fertilizer to sustain crop growth over many years on the same land. It was revolutionary, but I don't think the golden age is settled yet, even though some historians consider this era to have been it.

Equipment continued to develop with the proliferation of the diesel tractor. Tractors and implements made tilling, planting, cultivating, and harvesting much easier than it had been with coal-fired steam engines. Yields continued to increase as efficiency improved.

Then the modern era arrived. Technologies in plant varieties, pesticides, and even the often-maligned genetic modification pushed yields even higher while further reducing toil. Equipment continued to improve creating opportunities for farmers who were willing to take a risk.

So when was the golden age of farming? I believe it's today, and thirty-five years ago, and a hundred years ago, and two hundred years ago, and so on back to the dawn of civilization. After all, the quality and yields of both crops and livestock have not yet ceased to improve, and toil is constantly being reduced. Will the golden age continue? I have no doubt that it will.

WHAT IS FARMING?

That sounds like a silly question, but there's more to it than most may realize. I received a note recently from a college student majoring in music education. She said that, after graduation, she wanted to start a dairy farm and keep a small herd of happy cows to provide milk for the locals. I don't think she knew what she wished for.

Many of us have a romanticized notion of the farmer. We think of someone in bib overalls carrying a pitchfork looking after some cows and pigs while throwing scratch to the hens. It all seems so pastoral and serene. But just as there is a whole cast of characters that keeps the farm running smoothly, there is a lot more to the farmer's job than meets the eye. It's hard, dirty, sometimes unrewarding work. Its primary purpose is profit. It's a business, after all. Farming without the pursuit of profit is essentially gardening. In order to remain in existence, a farm has to at least break even. And there are a few things that any prospective farmer needs to know before breaking even can become a reasonable goal.

First, today's farming is *high-tech*. There is bovine genome sequencing, robots that milk cows, self-driving tractors, and genetically modified plants. Even a recent college graduate who just wants to milk a few cows for the locals won't be able to escape high technology.

Other careers are high-tech and sophisticated, like neurosurgeon or rocket scientist. But farming is complicated in a different way as the farmer must wear many hats. I'm not talking about a dusty ball cap with a seed logo or cowboy hat either. The term "factory farm" has a negative connotation, but in a sense, farmers indeed are like factory managers. They have incredible responsibilities to their families, employees, their livestock, the land and, ultimately, the food consuming public. Farms have many, many moving parts, both figuratively and literally, and the farmer keeps them moving together in concert like a symphony. You might not want a dairy farmer operating on your brain, but I wouldn't want a brain surgeon raising my food either.

Today's dairy cow is a sophisticated animal in her own right. This is not your great-grandfather's cow. No, she is built for performance. And that performance means producing milk by the bucketload. Today's lactating dairy cow, on average, needs to eat as much energy, pound for pound, as a person would need to run a marathon. And she eats mainly forage that is indigestible to humans. The average dairy cow does this every day, and the above average ones need even more energy. Getting the ration right for a high-producing dairy cow requires a bit more than a calculator and a note pad. It takes sophisticated computer programs, years of experience, and some instinctual cow-sense. Most dairy farmers employ the skill of a good bovine nutritionist, well acquainted with the latest technology, to get the job done.

Today's farming is inherently *risky*. There are times when I wonder if farmers would have a better chance if they just took the deed of the farm to Atlantic City and bet it all on a single hand of blackjack. But the farmers I know are highly skilled and not afraid of a little risk. In fact, it sometimes seems like they know how to count cards and beat the odds. Farmers are risk managers; they overcome broken equipment, government regulations, and even bad weather.

Today's farming is very *competitive*. If you aren't competitive, don't aspire to be a farmer. Yes, farmers are always willing to lend a hand to a neighbor, even when their help isn't requested. Competition among farmers is more a matter of pride than trying to eliminate other farmers from the playing field. Many compete to be the first one with corn planted in the spring, or to have silage (fermented livestock fodder) that yields and tests the best. Some compete to see who has the best cow at the show, and other farmers compete to lock up some rented farm ground. Farming is better for everybody with a little bit of competition.

Today's farming is *expensive*. Milking happy cows for the locals may be a laudable endeavor, but you might go broke before the end of one lactation cycle. Milking equipment can cost hundreds of thousands of dollars, and functional milk-cooling equipment is right there with it. Feed for dairy cows isn't cheap either, and it's not a one-time cost. Cows eat every day.

Today's farming is *thankless*. Farmers are, for the most part, not rich and famous. They don't have annual awards and I can't remember any reality shows about them. In fact, farmers are often, ironically, the subject of criticism from environmental groups and animal activists, despite being on the forefront of environmental steward-ship and animal welfare. With all of the difficulties in-volved in farming, why would anyone in his or her right mind want to do it?

Because today's farming is *essential*. The survival of civilization literally depends on it. Indeed, without farmers and modern farming practices we would face mass starvation; today's civil and political dramas would look like child's play by comparison. Some say the Arab Spring revolutions of 2011 and 2012 were caused by Middle Eastern grain shortages. There are historians who blame the fall of the Roman Empire on a deadly cattle virus called rinderpest. Farmers, despite the challenges they face, are an integral part of what makes a stable civilization possible. They provide *food security*.

FARMERS MAKE IT LOOK EASY

Growing food is hard.

To those of us who work in agriculture, it seems that Hollywood and other elements of the media are sometimes overly critical of the way farmers practice their profession. From common husbandry practices like dehorning and feed additives, to cropping technologies like fertilizers and pesticides, agriculture is the subject of excessive scrutiny.

As I drive down the back roads, I see field after field of crops that are in various stages of maturity. The crops are uniform, the rows are straight, and the yields are going to be good. Mother Nature deserves some of the credit for the yields, but the straight rows and uniformity fall squarely on the farmer.

Farmers make it look easy.

The vast majority of the population doesn't understand the pitfalls, challenges, and risks that farming involves. Maybe farmers make it look *too* easy. I always cringe when a commercial portrays a farmer as a toothless, straw hat-wearing hayseed unable to form a complete sentence. American farmers successfully fend off starvation for the three hundred million or so inhabitants of our country, including those who label them as country bumpkins.

Our country's food supply is wholesome, inexpensive and, most importantly, plentiful. Any civilization where obesity is a bigger problem than hunger is doing something right, and we have farmers to thank for that.

Good food doesn't come from taking shortcuts. Farmers tend to do things the hard way, and yet farm productivity increases every decade. Technology plays a role in this success, but farmers are really good at the behind-the-scenes work of putting it all together. Unfortunately, few of us get to appreciate the complexity of it all.

Husbandry practices like dehorning, castration, tail docking, and feed additives are not shortcuts. They have specific purposes and indications. Dehorning prevents injuries. Castration of steers reduces aggression and improves carcass quality. Tail docking, while controversial, does result in cleaner dairy cows. Feed additives allow the animals to utilize feed more efficiently, which decreases how much feed the animal needs.

Pesticides prevent crop failures caused by insects and other pests and reduce the amount of land necessary to grow the totality of our crops, including the roughly forty percent of our nation's corn that is grown for ethanol production. Genetically modified, or GMO, crops greatly reduce the amount of chemical pesticides that have to be applied, and they further reduce acreage necessary for farming, allowing more land to be set aside for wildlife habitat. There are no shortcuts.

I've been told that the only way to tolerate the long hours and the sometimes impossible business climate is if farming is in your blood, and there's no doubt in my mind that it's true. It's not a job; it's a calling. And while it's certainly not all doom and gloom, the work is hard and the conditions are often brutal. If there weren't rewards, nobody would be willing to farm. But since there are farmers, there must be good reasons for their choice of vocation.

Some might think that subsequent generations continue to farm out of tradition. That may be true in some cases, but I have known many farmers who have tried following in their parents' footsteps for the sake of saving the farm only to realize that it wasn't in their blood. And a few of my veterinary clients are first-generation farmers, so tradition isn't the only answer.

None of us really know what's in the minds of others, except maybe our spouses. (My wife has the uncanny ability to read my mind.) So the true motivation of farmers may never really be known. But I have a few ideas.

The motivation for profit certainly cannot be ignored. While the profit incentive is always present, the profits, unfortunately, are not. Maybe it's the lure of working outside that draws people to farming. In the spring, when the weather is nice and the grass is green, I absolutely love working outside. But in my part of Pennsylvania, where the winter lasts about nine months, that short stretch of nice spring weather may not be enough incentive.

Then there are people who just like a challenge. Maybe it's a form of stubbornness. I have a little of that streak in me. When I was contemplating going to veterinary school, people told me how hard it was. It motivated me all the more. If you want to convince a farmer to do something, tell him he can't do it. Then watch it get done.

And it can't be denied that there is a certain satisfaction in a job well done. Farmers take a lot of pride in doing things well and feel embarrassed when that one corn field that's visible from the road doesn't look good. They also take great pride in producing quality livestock. Genetic selection and raising quality stock isn't just a source of pride, it's a source of income.

The honest truth is that I don't know why farmers do what they do, but I'm grateful. And if my kids have farming in their blood, I won't dissuade them.

The perpetual challenge for farmers is to grow plentiful, affordable, and wholesome food year in and year out. Make no mistake, it is a challenge. Farmers, despite having to deal with equipment breakdowns, disease outbreaks, uncooperative weather, adverse business conditions, and countless other difficulties continue to rise to the occasion every year. And they always make it look easy.

THESE GUYS ARE GOOD

Since only about two percent of our population are farmers, that leaves the other ninety-eight percent dependent on them to grow the food that we enjoy. Be it meat, grains, or fruits and vegetables, farmers do the heavy lifting so the rest of us can relax a bit. These guys are good.

While most farmers aim to do right by the land, their livestock, and the food-consuming public, they also operate in the pursuit of profit in a very challenging market. Farmers have little control over what price they are paid for their product. Farmers who sell directly to the public are exceptions, but they are in the minority.

Instead, prices are set by the commodity markets. Farm products are commodities in the truest sense, meaning corn or beef or milk from one farm is indistinguishable from that of another farm. Profit is only realized through being more *efficient* than the competing farms. In order to be profitable, farmers must be efficient. This efficiency is reflected in the ever-increasing yields realized in both crops and meat and milk. As farms become more efficient, profit margins shrink. This is great for consumers, not so much for the farmers' bottom line. Yes, most farmers are particularly frugal and those that aren't usually end up in bankruptcy. One theme that is always in the minds of farmers is getting the best bang for the buck.

Most farmers are faced with tough efficiency decisions nearly every day. When a new medicine comes on the market for their cattle, the first question I, as a veterinarian, am asked is, "Is it worth the cost?" When a new crop is considered, they investigate to determine if it's better to pay a third party to conduct the harvest or to buy a new piece of equipment that can complete the harvest. When contemplating an expansion, they determine if it is more or less profitable than remaining static.

This efficiency is reflected in what we pay for our food. In the United States, only about ten percent of our household expenditures is used for food, with half of that being spent on restaurants and snack food. In that respect, we are the envy of the world.

No one is perfect and farmers are no exception. Just as in any other field, there are farmers who are unscrupulous, who find ways to circumvent the laws, or who mistreat their animals but by and large, farmers truly care about the well-being of their livestock. I know this because I have access to something that the general public rarely sees: the day-to-day operations of farmers, especially dairy farmers, who rise at four a.m. seven days a week to feed the cattle, milk the cattle, bed the cattle, and tend to the sick cattle. The public doesn't get to see the hundreds of millions of cattle, sheep, and hogs that are well treated, and never abused, every single day.

Time after time, farmers who would rather realize an economic loss than cause an animal to needlessly suffer call me, the veterinarian, to do the right thing. Be it patching up a sick animal or euthanizing one that is too sick for slaughter, farmers bear the financial cost of the just decisions they make. Standards in animal care have improved to the point that it can become truly economically burdensome for some farmers. Nonetheless, the vast majority continue to meet or exceed the standards.

Farmers are good at what they do. Good enough that we all trust them to provide us with something that none of us could survive without: our food.

AND SO ARE THE GALS

I started veterinary school a long time ago. One of my professors, in the middle of a lecture, used the term *dairyman*. Then he paused and added, "...and dairywomen too. You know, there are women dairy farmers and some of them are quite good at it."

Well, maybe he wasn't a hundred-percent politically correct, but the truth is, at the time, I hadn't considered that a woman could be a farmer. I didn't know any female farmers, and the idea that women could be farmers just wasn't the picture that had been drawn for me.

Of course, I now know better. They eventually let me graduate and I became a bona fide veterinarian. In my first job, I encountered dairywomen. They were quite skilled. My professor had been right, and I changed my concept of what a farmer could be.

Today, many of our dairy clients are women. Some are partners with their husbands in the farm, and others are on their own. Some are employed by the farm as herd managers or calf specialists. Drive around during planting season and you will no doubt see women driving tractors plowing fields, planting crops, and making hay.

Real life has a way of turning a stereotype on its head. Women play major roles on farms across the country. They milk the cows, feed the calves, and participate in the crop work. They are farmers in every sense of the word. Indeed, some of the hardest working people I've met anywhere are dairy women. Rise at three a.m. and milk the cows. Tend the children and/or grandchildren. Feed the calves. Make lunch. Tend the children. Milk the cows. Feed the calves. Make supper. Repeat.

I could generalize for a bit about the distinguishing characteristics of women versus men on the farm, but that's not the point. There is one characteristic that farm women possess, though, that I don't think anyone, dairyman or dairywoman, would deny: It's their ability to *nurture*.

Nurturing is important for any area of the farm. Cows, children and crops, among other things, require some degree of nurturing, but without doubt, the job requiring the most nurturing ability is raising the dairy calves. Dairy farmers, for the most part, hand raise their replacement heifer calves. It's better for both the calf and the cow since it reduces the transmission of disease, but the job requires a special degree of nurturing and patience. Sorry guys, but I think the ladies have us beat in that department. I've long held that if a farm is dissatisfied with the way their calves are growing, get someone's mom to raise them.

Farming stereotypes are not adequate descriptors of what's really going on in the barnyard. Farmers are many things. They are workers, businessmen, husbands and fathers. They are also wives, mothers, and women who take their jobs seriously and do them exceptionally well.

IT'S A TOUGH JOB . . .

I doubt that you could find more than a handful of people who don't agree that farmers are a hard-working bunch. The college student who dreamed of milking happy cows was exactly right about one thing: Like most other segments of society, farming has become quite specialized. Farmers tend to produce the product that suits them best, like meat, milk, or crops. They pick one thing and do it well. I know of only one farm that produces crops, beef, milk, eggs, and pork, all under the same enterprise. While I have great respect for them, I sometimes wonder about their sanity.

Dairy farmers have earned my utmost respect. I don't mean to take anything away from the beef farmers or the crop farmers or the pig farmers; they all do an excellent job of growing affordable, wholesome food. But, in my opinion, it's the dairy farmer who has the most difficult job. In addition to working with the whole cast of specialists and technicians that we just talked about, the dairy farmer has to be many things all at once: a cow person, an agronomist, a diesel mechanic, a human resources manager and, most importantly, a businessperson.

Being in charge of a bunch of cows is a difficult job in and of itself, but the dairy farmer is in charge of *dairy* cows. The dairy cow is a diva if there ever was one. She is the most fragile and demanding 1,500-pound animal on the face of the Earth. She needs the most comfortable accommodations, the most nutritious feeds, regular foot trimming (like a manicure), and she absolutely, positively, without exception must be milked at least twice a day. And the dairy farmer *must* provide her with these or she won't make milk. You see, happy cows make the most milk. Unhappy cows don't. Farmers like happy cows.

So you have to keep them happy. Caring for the cows is a difficult job, but raising her food is no easy job either. When you drive around the country roads and see field after field of growing corn or alfalfa or soybeans, it's easy to think that it must be a simple job. Just throw some seed on the ground and let Mother Nature take her course, right? There is an awful lot of crops out there. How hard could it be?

I think the agronomist part of the dairy farmer would disagree. It takes skill, hard work, some good fortune, and cooperative weather. And all of those crops don't plant themselves, nor do they harvest themselves. Planting and harvesting is done with the help of some pretty high-tech equipment. And high-tech equipment can be as much of a demanding diva as a dairy cow. It likes to break down, usually during the peak of the harvest or planting. Many skilled dairy farmers can diagnose and fix the problem themselves, but as the equipment gets more sophisticated, they find themselves reliant upon the equipment technician, another addition to the cast of characters.

Since many dairy farms have grown larger, most farmers have had to hire outside labor. With this comes a whole new set of responsibilities previously unknown to the farmer. Making payroll, scheduling workers, and even providing housing and benefits adds to the dairy farmer's long list of responsibilities.

But it's the business aspect of dairy farming that's often the most difficult. I suspect that if dairy farmers wanted to be businessmen, they would have traded their work clothes for business suits and done it. But if a dairy farmer wants to stay in business, the farm must turn a profit. This means buying the right equipment to provide value to the farm; and making decisions about which seed corn to buy, which employees to hire, and which cows to sell. If the wrong decisions are made, it could result in financial ruin. The dairy farmer wears many hats. The stereotypical dusty ball cap is but one of them, and the business hat may be the least favorite, but it is arguably the most important one.

... AND IT'S A WAY OF LIFE

Farming has changed enormously in the last decades. The competition is tougher. The regulations are stricter. The profit is smaller. The farms are bigger. Farms are increasingly technical, specialized systems capable of growing more food for a growing population than farmers of past generations could ever imagine. Crop yields in the Corn Belt boggle the mind as they surpass 5 tons of corn per acre. Beef yields and quality grade on a finished steer have made tremendous improvements over just a couple of generations. Milk yield in dairy cattle is approaching supernatural territory. Farmers are very good at what they do and they're getting better every day. This transition is to the benefit of all of us through plentiful, wholesome and affordable food.

But one thing hasn't changed, and I pray it never will: Farming is more than a job; it's a way of life. I see it every day. Farming is a family enterprise as much as it is a business enterprise. The children learn at an early age about the day-to-day operations of a farm. It makes sense, though, since the children are raised right in the midst of the enterprise from which their livelihood comes.

As the children grow in age, their knowledge of the farm increases. 4-H meetings, days in the field, and morning and evening shifts feeding calves can provide more educational value than a four-year degree. Even on the large dairies with many employees, family involvement is the rule, not the exception. Employees are a vitally important part of any farm, yet without family, I doubt many farms would run as smoothly.

Farmers live this lifestyle to the fullest extent. Yes, there are activities off the farm that don't involve agriculture like sports, music, or vacations. Farmers are a quite a diverse group and have varying interests. Yet, many off-farm activities still involve agriculture. For many farm families, taking a vacation does not necessarily mean getting away from it all. It means packing up the cattle, beef or dairy, and heading across the state or

31

even the country to exhibit their cattle. Other opportunities to get away are visits to livestock or equipment auctions, tractor pulls, rodeos, and agricultural expos. And more than once, a honeymoon has been spent browsing equipment, or even other farms, in the East Coast farming mecca of Lancaster County, Pennsylvania (often accompanied by mild objections from the new bride, but only mild ones). Farming is pervasive and all-encompassing. Even when farmers aren't on the farm, the farm is still on their minds.

The current economic circumstances of agriculture in our country are nearly dire. Prices for most farm commodities, from milk to meat and corn to beans, are at or below the break-even point. But farmers go through these spells regularly and have come to expect them. Farms are getting bigger, and many older ones no longer exist. But the family farm will survive; I'd bet my career on it. And it will survive because farm families don't just invest their money in it; they invest their *lives*.

THE FARM: MORE FUN THAN DISNEY WORLD

The college student who wants to raise happy cows might have a more rewarding and instructive experience as an *agritourist*. It would certainly be less pricey and a lot less labor-intensive.

In fact, agritourism seems to be all the rage these days. From the classic movie *City Slickers* to the hot new trend of cow cuddling, some people without farming backgrounds are rightly enamored with agriculture.

But this interest could lead to some awkward situations. Farmers certainly don't lead sheltered lives, but what might be socially appropriate for non-farm folks could indeed offend the sensibilities of the hard-working farmer. For example, it would be best if an agritourist arrived on the farm and remained silent about some of the novel aromas experienced. Yes, to the unaccustomed nose it might result in a bit of a shock. Suburban nostrils do take some time to adjust to the country air. But walking around with one's hand over one's nose might lead the farmer to feel unloved. There is no shortage of smells on a livestock farm. Fermented silage, diesel fuel, and the ubiquitous manure (watch your step) all have signature aromas. To those of us who are accustomed to it, the smell is barely noticeable. For the newbie, it could be awful. Nevertheless, leave the clothespin at home. You'll get used to it before the tour ends.

If you see a tractor, and chances are pretty good that you will, don't plan on getting behind the wheel. Tractors today are sophisticated, highly technical machines. And they are expensive. Some of them cost many times the value of the farmer's house. You're more likely to get a tour of the house than a ride on the tractor.

You're also likely to see some cows. Don't worry, this is normal. But what isn't normal is to tell the farmer that the cows are skinny, especially if they are dairy cows. Dairy cows might look skinny to the untrained eye, but to those who know them, they look like dairy cows should: a little on the thin side. There's a reason we never see an old, fat dairy cow. Fat dairy cows just don't make much milk, and a dairy cow that doesn't make much milk ceases to be a dairy cow and becomes a beef cow.

And by no means should you tell the farmer that the beef cows are fat. Again, to the untrained eye, they may appear to be rotund, but they might just be in peak sale condition. If her ear tag number is 747, don't remind the farmer that it's the same number as the Boeing wide body.

If lunch is part of the tour package, I'd recommend against requesting the "vegetarian option" at chow time. Unless the visitor has a life-threatening allergy to meat, it would be like requesting the chicken dinner at a beef ranch. The livestock farmer, after all, depends on the sale of meat to pay the mortgage, the employees, the feed bill and, yes, the veterinarian. In the off chance that one actually does require the vegetarian meal, it probably won't be on the menu anyway. In that case, your best option would be to make nice with the farm dog.

Speaking of the farm dog, if you meet one, be kind. They are often hard-working critters, just like their masters, and they can be a highlight of any farm tour. But be warned: One of the farm dog's tasks is to protect the farmer's property. Some farm dogs can be right suspicious of strangers, especially ones that smell like the city. Eye contact is okay, but if the backs of your legs bear any resemblance to a cow, you might get to enjoy the herding experience. Don't worry, there is no additional charge for that.

FARM LIFE IS FOR THE DOGS

When it comes to the dogs, farm dogs are a special breed. Actually, they are *many* special breeds. The German Shepherd, the Border Collie, and the Great Pyrenees are just a few that claim to have farm dog at their cores. Even mutts take on the role of farm dog when asked.

Their tasks are many. Farm dogs act as a security system. They alert the farmer when a stranger is snooping around the farm or when the delivery truck shows up with parts. Farm dogs protect the young stock from hungry coyotes. And they fend off hordes of hungry skunks on a quest for free cat food. Most farmers would rather feed a mooching skunk than have their canine get into a funky mess, but farm dogs are more than willing to take one for the team.

A good farm dog loves to patrol for groundhogs. After snatching one out of the field, the farm dog might bring it home for a measure of approval from his farmer. Once he receives a pat on the head, the good farm dog is likely to go and hide his spoils for few days. By that time, the fermenting groundhog carcass becomes an effective cover scent to conceal his dog essence, or skunk essence as the case may be.

Farm dogs live under the open sky. You won't find a farm dog curled up in bed with his farmer, even if it was allowed to be. Some farm dogs choose to sleep under the stars in the dead of winter even though the barn door is always open to them.

The Australian Cattle Dog, also known as a *heeler*, is arguably the toughest dog a farmer can get. Not very big, and tougher than a pine knot, these farm dogs are known to have more lives than a cat. I once saw one get hit by a car. It just got up, shook it off, and looked at me as if to say, "That didn't hurt!"

Heelers are named for a particular tendency they have. To get a cow to move, they bite at its heel, hence the name *heeler*. Cows kick pretty hard. I know; I've been the recipient of more than a few light feet. So when a heeler takes an instinctive chomp at a cow's heel, the cow levies an instinctive boot at the dog's chops. If the cow lands a hoof, the heeler gets an expression on his face that says *Is that all you got?*

You can almost read the heeler's mind when a cow is near. "Can I bite her heel? Can I bite her heel? Can I bite her heel? Please? Oh, *please?*" But the well-trained heeler waits for the command before proceeding. It really wants to bite at the cow's heel, but some will settle for just making the threat. If a farmer has a cow he wants to move and she's being obstinate, which cows are known to be sometimes, he can simply ask the heeler to bark. The mere bark of a heeler can make a down cow suddenly rise.

I've never owned a heeler, not because I don't like them, I just doubt that I could offer it enough fulfillment to keep it out of trouble. They like to work, and they can get a little neurotic without a full-time gig. In fact, they could become neurotic enough to find a heel, *any* heel, and chomp on it.

Dogs are happy by nature, but farm dogs are happiest when there is business to conduct. Running off skunks, exterminating groundhogs, terrorizing coyotes, and moving cows are labors of love. They are offered as much dog food as they want, but they choose more exotic fare when it's available. They have shelter, but prefer wide-open spaces. Farm dogs are rough around the edges and they live life fully. They are a special breed indeed, even though they are, in fact, many breeds.

CLEARING THE FIELD

Many livestock farms produce their own feed crops, adding a whole dimension of labor to an already busy mixture. The first step, before fertilizing and planting, is to clear the field, otherwise known as *picking up rocks*. Rocks can damage equipment and reduce crop yield, so they have to be removed. When I was a kid, this was the job I hated most (and believe me, there was a lot of competition).

You would think that picking up rocks and throwing them in a wagon, year after year, in the same field, would eventually eliminate all the rocks. On the contrary, it seemed that every year there were even more rocks that must have migrated up from the depths of the earth. To this day, if I never pick up another rock, it will be too soon.

Picking rocks, of course, isn't the only difficult farm job. Baling hay is, unquestionably, difficult work. Most guys who grew up in farm country have had the pleasure of baling the hay, loading it on a wagon, and then unloading it into a barn. It's hot, dusty, and the dry, stemmy grass makes your forearms look like hamburger after tossing only a few bales. Many farms have taken to baling at least a portion of their hay into large round or square bales. It saves a lot of work, but you lose the character-building aspect of stacking the forty-pound bales in a barn on a hot day in August.

I learned first-hand that building a fence is perhaps the single most demanding job on the farm. My wife is a goat farmer. In order to prevent the goats from wandering off, and also to prevent the coyotes from eating her goats, we needed a fence, so I fenced in about two acres.

I was able to borrow a post pounder from a friend of mine. The post pounder, as its name implies, pounds the post into the ground using the hydraulics from a tractor. But even with this labor-saving device, the person running the pounder can take quite a beating. Fifty-pound locust posts need to be pounded over and over again to set them two and a half feet into the ground, below the frost line.

My dad helped me set the posts one afternoon. He mentioned several times how much work the post pounder saved. When he was a kid, he used to set posts with a shovel and a post-hole digger. A friend of mine just fenced in a hundred acres to keep his cattle where they belong. I think I'd rather sell the herd.

But I'm getting ahead of myself. Clearing rocks is no fun and there's no easy way to do it. Pick them up, throw them in the wagon, and do it again next year.

POOP STINKS: MORE ABOUT MANURE

Poop. It's a dirty subject and a fact of life. It's an even bigger fact of life on farms since livestock are quite proficient at producing it. Dairy cows, in fact, can produce well over a hundred pounds of the green stuff a day (and yes, it's green). Even people who don't know much about farming know that poop is used for fertilizer (and I've already heard the "you are what you eat" jokes), but it doesn't get spread on the fields by itself. First it must be managed, and that's a whole experience unto itself.

I make my living at the rear ends of cows so, as you might imagine, I tend to be a poop magnet. Hardly a night goes by that my daughter doesn't ask me, "Daddy, do you have cow poop on you?" When I invariably say, "Yep" she gives me the usual "EWWWW!"

Cows that graze on fresh grass are the most likely to take aim and splat. Lush grass, as opposed to hay, doesn't have much substance. When the cow is finished with it, it has even less. A precarious place to be is behind a cow after she returns from pasture. If she decides to cough... well, I've learned not to stand too close to a cow's rear if she has a cough. Experience is the best teacher.

Since I am a poop magnet, my truck's interior also has the same magnetism. While I am very careful to change coveralls and to disinfect my boots between farms, the interior of my truck nonetheless bears the brunt of my occupation. Happily, someone got me a pine scented air freshener for Christmas, which means that the inside of my truck now smells like a cow pooped under a pine tree.

When I was in veterinary school, I had my first experience with getting poop in my eye. Being quite familiar with manure's composition, you could say I was worried about the future state of my eyesight. So when I asked my professor if I should be concerned, he told me that it was a rare day that he wasn't the recipient of the "poop in the eye" trick and he could still see just fine. As it turns out, it was a preview of my future vocation. And, yes, my eyesight is still fine.

Even though I can be splattered from head to toe and not give it a second thought, I still haven't reached the point where I can eat a sandwich unless my hands are clean. Several unexplained intestinal diseases and one explained intestinal infection have left me with a grave concern about eating with dirty hands. In fact, cow poop is known to contain several pretty nasty bugs including salmonella and E. coli. I don't take those lightly. Clients may tease me ("Come on, it's only grass and water"), but I always wash my hands before I eat.

Yes, it stinks, causes stains, and can potentially make a person sick, but it's also pretty useful stuff. It even has recreational value. The Iowa State fair has an annual cow chip-tossing contest, not to be confused with the cow *pie*-tossing contest which is a little messier.

But seriously, manure does have some legitimately redeeming qualities. It makes excellent fertilizer. Not only does it add nutrients like potassium, phosphorus, and nitrogen to the soil, it also returns much needed organic material necessary for water retention and other functions. Throughout the year, manure on dairy farms is gathered and stored in tanks or pits that are emptied as one of the first steps to prepare for spring planting. It's the beginning of the process of growing the crops that will sustain the farm for the next year. Most dairies have the capacity to store manure for about six months in a pit or tank that prevents leeching into the ground. In the spring and fall, they get emptied out and spread on the fields. Some smaller farms don't have any storage capacity for manure. Since we can't ask the cow to stop pooping, those farms have to spread their manure on the fields as fast as it is produced regardless of how harsh the weather conditions are.

But those farms that do have the ability to store manure get their share of dirty looks from neighbors and passersby in the early spring when they empty their tanks. And farmers know how unpleasant it can be to drive behind the manure truck after it has spread its payload, but it has to be done. The bottom of your vehicle may get a new layer of undercoating (now green) and become the object of curiosity of every dog in the neighborhood.

Every spring, the first step in growing crops is to apply a good coat of manure. It's not like the farmers are sadistic and want to ruin the day for everyone who's driving around the back roads, but manure application is a necessary evil. Please believe me when I state that it is indeed necessary to "stir the pot" and let the "poop hit the fan." Liquid manure that's been in the storage tank for months smells like rotten eggs on sauerkraut, and before it's loaded onto the tank spreader it has to be agitated. Try to avoid being downwind of the storage pit when that happens.

For those of you who have experienced the fresh country air in the springtime and felt compelled to proclaim something like, "There ought to be a law against that," as my very own mother has been known to say, I'd like to offer this tidbit: Getting rid of the stored manure and cleaning out the pens are perhaps two of the most unpleasant chores on the farm. The only thing that might be worse is picking rocks. But somebody has to do it. Consider yourself fortunate that you get to experience the effects from afar.

Herbivore manure makes excellent fertilizer not only because it replenishes the soil with nutrients like nitrogen and potassium, but also because it adds organic matter to the soil that helps retain moisture and builds topsoil. If you're lucky enough to live near a farm you may have noticed an unfamiliar odor, utterly unlike the typical herbivore manure fragrance, blowing in the wind. It has a particularly foul (or fowl) smell that might be useful as a tool for the enhanced interrogation of terrorists. The source of that funk is poultry manure and few things rival its peculiar aroma.

Poultry manure is usually brought into an area by truck from places that have large concentrations of chicken and turkey farming. It's relatively inexpensive and very high in nitrogen which is needed to give the crops a good start. I pity the truck drivers who have to haul it on the Interstate. I can only imagine the cursing and rude gestures they have to endure from the other drivers.

One of our neighbors procures a few loads of this brown gold every spring. One night, I was tipped off to this fact even before the wind shifted, bringing the definitive evidence to our door. I was on the porch as the empty spreader truck drove past our house. I braced myself for the shock. Wait for it... Wait for it...

UGGGGGHHHHH!!!!! Whoa, it's even worse than last year! Later that evening, as I was working in the house, the wind suddenly shifted and we were directly in the line of fire. It was warm that evening and the windows were open. Once that green fog drifted in, we dashed around the house sealing up any points of entry and regretting that we hadn't taken Homeland Security's advice to purchase plastic and duct tape.

Yes, thank goodness for spring. The fields turn green, the peepers serenade us, and the air is thick with the aroma of, well, spring. But without this process of recycling the manure to grow the crops, the very cycle of life couldn't be sustained.

It's unpleasant, but inevitable. It has to be spread. It does little good in the tank. In the field, it contributes to the growth of the corn, soybeans, alfalfa, or whatever feed crop is to be harvested. It adds organic matter back to the soil, enabling a fertile soil bed for generations.

In fact, if it isn't spread on the field, you know what will happen to it: It will follow the path of least resistance and will eventually find its way to the ocean by way of streams and rivers. That would make no one happy.

Yes, it stinks. It stinks, that is, until one becomes acclimated to the aroma. How long that takes is inversely proportional to the amount of exposure before about age ten. In other words, if you grew up with cow poop on your shoes, it doesn't stink for long. If you grew up in the city and find yourself five miles downwind of a cornfield, the acclimation process may take a month or two. Be glad this book doesn't come with scratch-and-sniff stickers.

And just when you hoped we were done talking about cow poop, here's one more thing: Before it becomes fertilizer, it might have been used to provide the cow a comfortable place to lay down. If organic bedding, like straw or wood shavings, is added daily to the cow's bedding area, the poop can be left to build up, and the packed manure provides good footing and a dry, comfortable bed. Some farms will agitate the bedding daily with a plow, causing the pack to compost, killing bacteria and reducing moisture. It even provides heat in the colder months. The cows remain clean and comfortable. Ironic, isn't it? Some larger farms will *digest* the manure to produce methane. The captured methane powers an electricity generator and the digested manure solids, once stable, will be used as bedding for the cows. If kept dry, it makes a comfy stall for the cows to lie down.

THE CYCLE OF CROPS

When I was younger, I marveled at the yearly cycle of farming. It all seemed so complicated. Planting and harvesting have to be done at the right times or the yield is poor and the crop is ruined. The weather has to cooperate too, but that's under the control of Providence.

The cycle still amazes me. The first step, as we just spent several paragraphs discussing, is to spread the manure. There is a multitude of ways that cow manure is stored and handled, but it all, eventually, makes its way back to the field. The chemical makeup of manure makes it an excellent fertilizer. It is rich in nitrogen, phosphorus, and potassium, all of which are necessary for plant growth. While spreading manure stinks, both literally and figuratively, it is an essential component of the cycle.

Once the manure is spread, the ground can be tilled under and the crops planted. Traditionally, the one of first crops to go in the ground is oats. Oats aren't exactly a cash crop, but because it provides shade it makes a good companion crop for alfalfa and grass which will become *hay*, or *silage*. Silage is forage that isn't completely dried and goes through a fermentation process, thereby maintaining the stability of the crop well after harvest. (Silage is kept in *silos*. Get it?) The oat straw that is left after harvest will be used for bedding.

After the oats are in, then the soybeans and the corn get planted. Of all the crops that the dairy farmer has, corn is probably the most critical. An early planting can result in an exceptional yield, but if the corn is planted *too* early the farmer runs the risk of losing the crop to a late frost.

By the time the corn and soybeans are in, the first crop of hay is ready to be baled or ensiled. Depending on the species of grass used for hay, if the harvest isn't done soon after the corn is in, the plant becomes too mature and the energy and protein content will drop substantially. Forage with low energy limits milk production. The protein can be replaced with grain supplementation, but it adds significantly to the farmer's feed bill.

So, after the crops are in the ground the farmer can relax, right? It would be nice, but no. Successive cuttings of hay need to be taken to harvest enough feed and to maintain quality. The crops need to be sprayed or cultivated to keep them from being eaten by pests or choked out by weeds. Just as manure happens, equipment breakdowns happen. Equipment must be maintained and repaired to keep the endless cycle of planting and harvesting on track.

The amount of feed it takes to feed 100 dairy cows in a year is 3,650,000 pounds or 1,825 tons. That's a lot of feed and a lot of exhausting work. So the next time you smell the aroma of spring in the air, recognize that it may stink for a couple of days, but it will soon make the crops green and healthy.

THE SECRETS OF SILAGE

As the end of summer approaches, the farmers' process of raising feed for their livestock nears its end. It began late in the winter, when the seed that would eventually become this year's crop was delivered, progressed through field preparation, manure spreading, planting, pest control, and sometimes even irrigation. The small grains, alfalfa and any other feed crops have been harvested leaving only the corn, the last crop in the ground.

This corn crop is destined to become corn silage, the staple of a dairy cow's diet. There are certain parameters that should be satisfied for the corn plant to be ready for harvest, or *chopping*. First, the corn grain itself should be in the process of maturing. When the top of the corn kernel starts to dent, it is becoming mature and is almost ready for harvest. Second, when the moisture content of the chopped plant falls to about sixty-five percent, it's time to chop. If corn is chopped too wet, much of the extra water will run off during the packing process, robbing the corn silage of many of its valuable nutrients. On the other hand, if the moisture content is too low, the chopped plant may not pack tightly enough, letting in air and causing molding and spoilage.

Chopping the corn is merely the first of many steps in the crop's journey to become fermented feed for cattle. Once chopped, the corn may receive an inoculation of beneficial bacteria to aid fermentation, which is required to stabilize the product and prevent rot. Farmers used to rely solely on the bacteria found in the soil to ferment the corn. Some still do, but there are species of bacteria not native to the soil that have superior characteristics for fermenting silage. These are commercially available for application during chopping.

Some farmers may add preservatives, like proprionic acid, to ensure an even more stable silage. Proprionic acid is naturally produced by bacteria during the fermentation process, adding more further increases stability.

Whether treated with additives or not, once chopped, the next step is packing. This must be done immediately after chopping or the chopped plant may begin to heat rapidly and destroy the feed. If corn silage is put into a tall upright silo, gravity does the work of packing, freeing up the farmer's time for other jobs. If, however, the silage is to be stored in long trench silos, it has to be actively packed. This is where some really big, heavy tractors are needed. As a load is dumped on the pile, it has to be spread out evenly and driven over again and again to ensure a good pack. Packing eliminates much of the air from the silage, allowing the fermentation process to start. It's like the opposite of composting, in which decay is the whole point.

The next step is the actual fermentation. If packed properly, all available oxygen is consumed by the microbes during the initial phase and then there is a transition to anaerobic fermentation. As the anaerobic bacteria continue to consume the plant's sugar for energy, they release acids, eventually producing enough acid to bring about their own demise. So, once the bacteria have "pickled" themselves to death, a new batch of silage is born. It is actually way more complicated than that, but I think you get the basic idea. Silage is sort of like sauerkraut, but not made from cabbage.

The fermentation process takes a minimum of two weeks to result in a stable silage, although most bovine nutritionists recommend waiting for about a month, if possible, before disturbing it. Like a fine wine, as silage ages, its quality improves. But if fermentation was altered, due to inadequate packing or not enough moisture, for example, its quality will deteriorate over time.

A farmer several years ago told me that he had finally reached some corn silage at the bottom of the silo that was put up in 1978. It looked good, smelled good, and the heifers who ate it that day thought it tasted good. It had obviously gone through a good fermentation process or it would have transformed into compost long ago. In 1978, Jimmy Carter was president, the Pittsburgh Steelers had only won two Super Bowls and I was only... well, let's just say that I was much younger, and that batch of silage was better preserved than I am.

NOT YOUR GRANDPA'S FARM

The image of the family farm with some beef cows, dairy cows, chickens, pigs, and horses is comforting. The family farm still exists—it's estimated that of all farm enterprises in the United States, about 98% are family owned—but it's no longer our grandfather's family farm.

In agriculture, as in many other industries, there has been a steady trend towards specialization and consolidation. There are fewer farms today, and they are bigger than the ones of the past. They also tend to specialize in one area of production like crops, dairy, beef, or hogs. It can be difficult to accept sometimes, but those involved in agriculture can attest that unless you adopt new technology and superior management practices, the prospects for running a profitable operation decrease. That doesn't mean that the adage "get big or get out" is true; on the contrary, there are many very successful small farms today that can support a family. But the small farm must be run very well to survive. I spend most of my time on farms that have chosen to focus on dairy production which means that, every day, I have the opportunity to get up close and personal with that noble, majestic beast, *the cow*. Let's pull back the curtain and reveal this amazing creature in all of her glory . . .

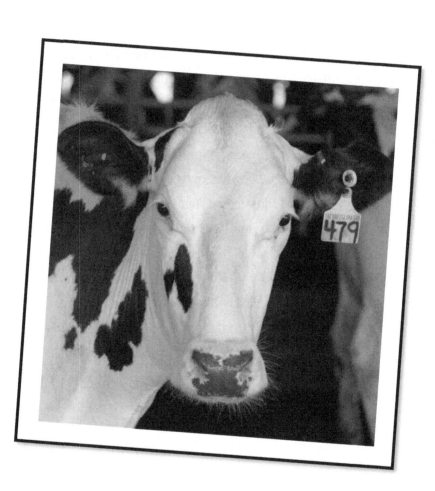

Part Two
THE MAJESTIC COW

God made every kind of wild animal, every kind of tame animal, and every kind of thing that crawls on the ground. God saw that it was good. Genesis 1:25

I know that the universe is ordered to a purpose from the most distant galaxy to the closest organism that exists in a commensal relationship with man. My faith tradition teaches it and I accept it. But sometimes I don't comprehend exactly why.

Could God have done it differently, maybe without animals? He certainly could have. Humans are created in His image and likeness while animals are not. Nevertheless, He found the animals to be "good" and the entirety of His creation to be *"very* good." Indeed, the existence of animals, especially those which have been domesticated, is good and makes our lives better than if we had to live without them.

Farm animals provide products upon which humanity literally depends. The greatest of these, perhaps, are meat and milk. Could we survive on plants alone? We could, but human civilization would likely be a lot different if plants were our only option to eat. For people, animal proteins are akin to superfood. It's energy dense and contains essential nutrients like certain amino acids, fats, and minerals that are in plants, but at far lower levels.

Consider also that ruminants, such as cattle and sheep, thrive on plants that are largely indigestible to humans. Ruminants can unlock the energy from within the cell walls of plants and convert it into meat and milk which feeds, in a very efficient manner, human beings. The animals do most of the work and the humans reap the benefits. This is important since the majority of the ruminant's life is spent eating forage as opposed to grains. I don't believe this planet could sustain its seven-plus billion people without some help from ruminants.

Clothing, in the form of leather and wool, are durable, protective, and insulating for people of many climates. The amazing cotton plant notwithstanding, there are few plant-based substitutes for these animal products.

Animals have been used for draft for millennia and they continue to provide labor in many parts of the world. Horses and oxen are capable of providing power that we smaller humans can't rival. Even today, in the industrialized West, we measure the power generated from a machine by comparing it to a horse.

Animals create economic activity since they, along with their products, possess monetary value. This one hits me close to home since I make my living based on the income that animals provide for their farmers.

All livestock, including horses, can provide leisure. Competitive events like rodeo and livestock judging entertain rural and city folks alike. There are also those who raise livestock, ride horses, or keep sheep for wool purely for enjoyment.

And I haven't even mentioned the companion animals. The human-animal bond is very real and has been the subject of extensive study. Our culture considers the pet to be as much a part of the family as the children.

I gave my dog some scratch behind the ears one day and he truly dug it. He's a Golden Retriever and he is a *really* good dog. I'm sure your dog is good too, but not as good as mine. He looked into my eyes and I wondered what on Earth he could be thinking about. He wasn't contemplating the cosmos or thinking about his Creator. I still don't know what he was thinking because, while he is a *really* good dog, he still can't talk.

When I held both of my children for the first time, I was both awestruck and filled with an overwhelming sense of responsibility. Our relationships with our children and family are, or should be, a mirror of the love God has for His children. It's way more than a pet can provide. Nonetheless, when I gave my dog some scratch that day, I was grateful for him. I was grateful for his existence and the enjoyment he brings to our family. I am hardly alone in this sentiment. Maybe God created animals as further evidence that He loves us and wants us to be happy.

One summer day, while on my way to doctor a sheep, I watched a large black bird with a majestic white head and white tail feathers, glide along the river valley. *Wow*, I thought, *a bald eagle. I haven't seen one of those in years.* One of the perks of my job is the opportunity to observe the various wildlife that live in my neck of the woods.

The bald eagle is an incredible animal and I laud the folks who decided generations ago that it should be our national bird. Legend has it that Benjamin Franklin wanted it to be the turkey. Thankfully, common sense prevailed.

I can't help but reflect upon the majesty of God's many creatures. There's the whitetail deer that, despite its hazard to motorists, is also beautiful and majestic. The

Superman of the wilderness, the deer can leap with incredible agility and seemingly outrun a speeding bullet. And if the privilege of glimpsing one isn't enough, the hunter who has the good fortune to harvest one or two is rewarded yet again with sustenance for the long winter months.

And there's the comedian of the woods, the squirrel. Describing squirrels as *hyperactive* doesn't come close to doing them justice; it's far more accurate to say that they're hyperactive with a triple espresso. Up and down, back and forth, in search of the elusive nut, they are majestic in their own industrious way, entertaining those who wait patiently for a glimpse of the elusive whitetail deer.

There are countless other majestic forest creatures, like the turkeys, the hawks, and the foxes. They're nice, but I'd be willing to bet that when God created the birds and the land animals, he must have been especially satisfied with one of them in particular: *the cow.*

I don't know when wild cows roamed the Earth, but I wish I could have been there to see it. Yes, I readily admit my bias. The cow is more than just another of God's creatures to me; she is my livelihood. Whether it's fixing her when she's broken, helping the farmer make her more productive, or trying to replicate her, the cow helps me feed my family. And she is the same to many other veterinarians, hoof trimmers, artificial breeders, and, of course, farmers around the world.

When God made the cow, He must surely have realized that she is something special. I'd reckon that's why she's so important to humans. God created humans to know and love Him, but he must have created the cow to provide for us.

She provides income for the farmer. She provides a challenge for the veterinarian. She provides meat for all of us, along with multitudes of dairy products. She provides leather for clothing and industry and countless other uses.

She is also very green. Her complex digestive system enables her to graze grass that is indigestible to humans, allowing farmers to produce her food without tilling up the soil. She has also been known to consume that which is considered waste by the rest of us, like citrus pulp, beet pulp, soybean hulls, distillers grains, and many other byproducts that would otherwise be put in a landfill to rot.

She is bound by the chains of instinct, but still has personality. Cows have been present throughout recorded human history, a true partnership for the ages. Did humans domesticate the cow, or did cows domesticate humans? My bet is on the latter. She isn't as nimble as the whitetail deer, and she isn't as grandiose as the bald eagle, but she is nonetheless majestic, and more important to humanity than any animal of the forest.

BARNYARD TOP TEN:
THE WIDE, WIDE WORLD OF COWS

Cows are like family to me. I spend most of my waking hours in their company. I probably see more of them than I do my own family. That's okay. I love my family, but cows can't talk, a trait which makes them great listeners. I can say whatever I want and the cow will only nod and silently agree. At least that's what I like to think they do. If I'm being honest, it's more likely that they're counting the minutes until I shut up and leave. If only cows could tell time.

Over the course of my career I've become pretty familiar with the many idiosyncrasies of cows, and I've grown rather fond of them. If you've spent quality time with our pasture-dwelling friends, I have no unique insights to offer. But for those of you who know cows only from the other side of the fence, here's a ten-point orientation to help you get acquainted with their many charming quirks.

10. COWS ARE CURIOUS. Curiosity may have killed the cat, but it usually only gets the cow in trouble. When farmers let the cows out of the barn after milking time, they have to investigate everything from the empty bag on the walkway to the strange person in green coveralls (me) waiting for them to leave.

9. COWS ARE IRRITABLE. Yes, the docile cow has an irritable side. Just ask her to stand still for a moment so that I can examine a part of her, like maybe inside her rear end, and you'll get acquainted with the grouchy side of the cow.

8. COWS DEMAND THAT YOU RESPECT THEIR PERSONAL SPACE. Scientists refer to a cow's personal space as her *flight zone*. When you approach a cow in the field, she will let you get close, but not too close. The tamer she is, the closer you can get, but if you intrude too much she will back away. If she is tethered in a stall and can't flee, she still has a flight zone, but she reacts differently if you intrude on her. Almost universally, if you place a hand anywhere on a tethered cow, she will lower head and shake it as if she's trying to get rid of the cooties you just gave her.

7. COWS HAVE MULTIFUNCTIONAL TONGUES. A cow's tongue is indispensable. More than just a fleshy eating utensil, she may use it to clean her nostrils or groom her back. She uses it to stimulate her newborn calf to breathe. She may use it to investigate that strange person who is trying to invade her flight zone. When she is bored, it becomes a toy. It has more uses than a Swiss Army knife.

6. COWS HAVE STRANGE DENTITION. Cows lack teeth on the upper part of the front of their mouth. Instead they have *dental pads*. The absent incisors are simply unnecessary to the cow and, for that matter, all other ruminants. As a grazer, the tongue does the grasping and pulling of the grass (yet another use!), literally wrapping around the vegetation and ripping it. They have no need to bite, and the fact that they are unable to do so is a legitimate reason for a veterinarian to decide to specialize in cattle. They also don't chew their food. Well, not at first. That would just delay the next bite of feed. But once the cow has eaten her fill, the chewing commences . . .

5. COWS CHEW CUDS. This also is common to all ruminants. Cows regurgitate and chew their cud, not to be a disgusting pig (sorry, pigs are not ruminants), but to extract every last bit of nutrition out of her meal. She breaks down the fibrous part of the plant with every chew, thereby releasing more of the good stuff like protein and sugar for digestion.

4. COWS DROOL. They drool a *lot*. It's been estimated that a cow can produce between twenty-five and fifty quarts of saliva every day. Cow saliva contains copious amounts of bicarbonate. It is the perfect buffer for her *rumen,* the large thirty to forty-gallon chamber of the cow's complex forestomach that ferments her food prior to digestion (Never heard of it? Don't worry; we'll talk more about it soon). This saliva buffer helps keep the rumen healthy. Most of it gets swallowed, but just watch any cow up close and you'll see the excess drool run out of her muzzle.

3. COWS BELCH. Cows burp a lot. They don't feel the need to excuse themselves because burping is just expected of them. As ruminants, the digestion process produces a lot of gas. Just like their salivary output, the volume of gas produced as part of the fermentation process is staggering, with estimates ranging from thirty to fifty quarts per hour. If a cow can't burp, she will literally die within a matter of hours, which is one reason why you'll rarely see a cow lying on its side. As relaxing as it may be, a cow who reclines on its side cannot burp, and a cow who cannot burp will eventually die from the accumulated pressure. The gas will build pressure in her rumen and cause her to bloat until she resembles a hot air balloon, except she won't be lighter than air.

2. COWS ARE ALLELOMIMETIC. There's a ten-dollar word for you. It means that cows like to mimic the behavior of other cows. When one cow goes outside, they all go outside. When one cow gets up to eat, they all get up to eat. When one cow lies down in the pasture, all of them follow and the fishing is bound to be poor... Oh, sorry, that's from a different list.

1. COWS MAKE GREAT HAMBURGERS. I know, it sounds harsh. But as much as I like cows, I always remember the reason for their existence. They provide food and fiber (leather) for humanity. In fact, given its long history of domestication and the many ways that it has supported human welfare and development, the cow could very well be the most important animal in all of human history.

Now that your high-level orientation is out of the way, let's mix in with the herd and get better acquainted with the charming traits that make cows so much fun.

CURIOUS COWS

Cats are curious. Get a new package delivered and the cat will investigate the inside of the box before moving in and claiming it as a new residence. Place a new house plant on the shelf and the cat will climb the wall to check it out. Put a new roll of toilet paper in the holder and you'll find it unrolled and piled on the floor within an hour. Cats just can't help themselves.

Indeed, curiosity would have killed more cats if it weren't for their nine lives, but when it comes to curiosity, the cat has nothing on the cow. One crucial difference: The stewardship of the farmer and the cautious nature of cows keeps them out of trouble most of the time. As soon as you step foot in a barn, the cows are compelled to investigate. They just can't help themselves. A group will approach you, but they'll stop within several feet to get a good look. Once they have surveyed the situation thoroughly, one cow will extend her head closer. Since she can't fully reach yet, she cautiously takes a step, then another, until she can just barely stretch out and feel you with her muzzle and get a good whiff through her nose.

Now, the cow makes a big decision. If you don't feel right to her muzzle, or even stink, she'll recoil in disgust, shake her head, clear her nostrils and retreat. If, on the other hand, you feel right or smell okay, she may investigate further. I still don't know what feels right or smells good to the cow. I'm trying to figure it out.

If you pass the first test, the taste test comes next. She will cautiously stick out her tongue for a quick lick. Cattle, like two-year-old children, do a lot of investigating with their mouths. You can't reason with a two-year-old child about the validity of the germ theory; neither can you reason with a cow. If it tastes bad, she bolts like lightning. If it doesn't taste bad, she may hang around for a little more until she tires of the experience. I also haven't figured out what makes a cow flee after disliking what she found with her tongue. I like to think I have a pleasant odor and taste, but the person is usually the last one to know, right?

If you have the opportunity (and permission), stand in the middle of a cow pasture sometime. Once the cows know you're there, you will be thoroughly investigated. The entire group will approach you, even if they have to walk a long way to get there.

Once, while I was treating a sick cow in the field, a cow approached me to investigate. All the while, unknown to me, the rest of the herd was hard at work investigating my truck. Fortunately, I've treated enough cows in the pasture to know that I need to keep the doors to my truck and workbox shut unless I want my stuff reorganized.

When I finished treating the sick cow, I learned that my truck was, in fact, not objectionable to the cows. They liked it. When I returned I found it coated in slobber and slime. Since cows eat off the ground, when the slobber and slime dried, it left a crust of dry mud on every square inch. It didn't look like I had gone four-wheeling, though, it was more like some kind of abstract art. I considered selling it to the Louvre and calling it *Cow Licked,* but I needed my truck later that day. So much for my career as an art mogul.

Calves are good at tongue investigations too, and their oral curiosity usually gets them in trouble. They don't believe me when I tell them about the germ theory, they just keep on licking, and they get a lot of gastrointestinal infections as a result.

Anyway, cows are curious by nature. And because cows don't have nine lives, farmers do their best to keep them out of trouble. A strategically placed electric fence, well grounded, can be a shocking discovery to a curious cow who wants to inspect the greener grass on the other side. Usually, the cow learns that the fence is off limits by her normal investigative prowess. She approaches, takes it in with her nostrils, and reaches out for a feel with her muzzle.

SNAP!

She rarely makes that mistake again.

And it's not just the greener grass on the other side of the fence that the farmer aims to protect. The farmer must also protect the cow from herself. If left to investigate fully, even though she is cautious, the cow is bound to get into trouble. There are such obstacles as frozen ponds in the winter that, while they look solid, can create a cowsicle within hours. The manure pit, while it looks like solid ground to the cow, instead acts like quicksand. And farm equipment is a cow magnet. While it looks benign, it offers nothing but trouble. The electric fence saves the cow from herself.

Cows will satisfy their curiosity, even if it's the last thing they do. It's a distinguishing characteristic. Ironically, the only thing they seem to never want to investigate is the barn cat.

CAUTIOUS COWS

Caution is the counterpoint to the cow's natural curiosity. While cows may be portrayed as brazen when they try to convince us to "EAT MOR CHIKIN," they are actually very careful. In fact, their wariness is one of their best-known attributes. Cows are so cautious that if there are any distractions in their path they will balk.

This distraction may be as minute as a piece of paper towel on the ground or an out-of-place tool. Even when running cows through a *working chute* (a gated path designed to move cattle from one place to another), they will stop to investigate anything that's out of place. Designing cattle working chute systems is an art and a science. If there are distractions, like a piece of paper on the ground, cow flow will bottleneck and the work grinds to a halt. Even a shadow will spook cows to the point that they refuse to move until it has been investigated and approved. The very best cattle chutes are designed to be boring so that the cows will move through as if a policeman were directing them, saying, "OK, move on now; nothing to see here."

When a cow is startled by an unfamiliar object or an unexpected event, they tend to overreact. When approaching a cow, one must always remember not to surprise her. A surprised cow will make a hasty retreat, and because cows are herd animals, the fear spreads to the other cows in her immediate vicinity. Within seconds the cows flee in terror. It's not exactly a stampede, but in their hurry to get away they may slip and fall and injure themselves, especially when they're on concrete.

COWS NEED GLASSES

When investigating alien objects, cows don't get up close and personal to get a good look. This brings up another attribute of the cow: poor eyesight. Admittedly, her eyesight might not actually be poor since she can spot an out-of-place item from a long distance, but her eyesight is different from yours and mine. A cow's eyes face 180 degrees away from each other on either side of her head. All prey species, including rabbits, sheep, and horses are like this. The widely separated eyes offer a broad field of vision and allow for early detection of a predator from any angle. Predator species, like dogs, cats, and even humans, have eyes that both face forward, allowing for depth perception. Cows lack depth perception, but they make up for it in discretion.

This lack of depth perception makes walking on uneven ground or negotiating a curve tricky for the cow. If she doesn't know how far the ground is from her foot, her cautious nature kicks in. Training a cow to walk onto a stock trailer, or to step up into an elevated pen, isn't a task for the impatient. When working with cows, patience is more than a virtue; it's a requirement.

COWS VALUE DIVERSITY

I know what you're thinking: *Cows have no concept of diversity.* You're probably right. Nonetheless, cows are diverse. There are beef cows and dairy cows, longhorn cows and hornless cows, and every kind of cow in between. There are cows with long ears and cows with short ears, cows that like cold weather and those who like hot weather, cows who have humps and those without, sacred

cows and edible cows. Yes, diversity really is a distinguishing characteristic of the cow.

COWS WORK HARD

One cattle characteristic to which many of us can relate is
hard-working. The dairy cow, when she is geared up to
make milk, works harder than anyone. Every day, she expends more energy than a marathon runner to produce her
milk. Some dairy cows are just plain workaholics. Gigi,
a Holstein cow in Wisconsin, recently set the record for
annual milk production: 74,650 pounds. For those of you
without calculators, that's just over twenty-three gallons
a day. How long would it take you to *drink* twenty-three
gallons of milk? Impressive indeed.

COWS ARE LAZY

I know, I just said that cows work hard, but I have a good
explanation for the contradiction. Cows love to lounge
around. In fact, it's good for them. After a big meal, a cow
will pick out a nice place to relax and chew on her cud.
Cud chewing allows her to be able to efficiently digest
the fibrous feed that is indigestible to simple-stomached
creatures like the pig or the dog.

This time spent lounging around is actually part
of her job. Imagine having a job like that! But it isn't just

to give her time to chew her cud. Lying down also improves blood flow to her udder, bringing nutrients that she needs to synthesize the various components of milk like lactose, fat, and protein. She gets more done by lounging than some people accomplish in an entire day.

COWS ARE LARGE . . .

Some cows are large, some are larger, and some are outright enormous. The average size of a milking Holstein (the famous black-and-white milk cow) is around 1,400 pounds. Some of the largest cows tip the scales at well over a ton. Combine the easily spooked nature of the cow with her large mass and she becomes an accident waiting to happen. She has tremendous inertia when she hits the deck.

But when not spooked, the cow tends to be slow and deliberate. Slow and steady wins the race to the milking parlor, the new pasture, or wherever the destination. Cows are bred for production, not speed.

. . . BUT THEY ARE NOT SMART

A wise man once told me that the only way a cow could be dumber is if she were bigger. It's true: Cows aren't very smart, but they don't really have to be. They have to be smart enough to eat and follow the herd. Anything beyond that would be overachievement, and cows are not ambitious.

I guess it is unfair to call them dumb; it is better said that they lack intelligence. Cattle are instinctual critters. Their basic instincts are twofold: find food and avoid *being* food. They do an excellent job at the former. Fortunately for the beef consumer, they are a dismal failure at the latter.

In my opinion, the degree of intelligence in an animal is inversely proportional to its instincts. Those of us who work with cattle use this to our advantage. Cows, while lacking intelligence, are still pretty easy to train, and to train cows, one must simply outsmart them. Seems like an easy enough task, right? It can be, but sometimes it isn't.

If we want a group of cows to be restrained together, to take blood samples, give vaccinations, or even perform pregnancy checks, we can induce them to cooperate by tempting them with tasty food. Some barns have self-locking head yokes. When the cow puts her head through the yoke to get a bite to eat, she trips a lever that closes a gate on her neck just tight enough to prevent her from withdrawing her head. Self-locking head yokes can restrain an entire group of cows at a time which also satisfies another instinct of the cow: to stay together as a herd. We can do this over and over again without the cows ever realizing that they're being tricked.

But once in a while, there comes along a cow that's smarter than the average cow. Some cows will figure out that if they don't put their head down all the way they can avoid getting caught. Let me tell you, it's no fun being outsmarted by a cow.

We can restrain individual cows for procedures in the same type of locking head yoke. Once, as I was collecting embryos from a restrained dairy cow, I noticed that she kept flicking her right ear. What I thought was a nervous tic was really a brazen escape attempt. The cow finally succeeded in releasing the latch by hitting it with her ear. I watched in speechless horror as she backed out of the restraint, her indwelling catheter still connected to the collection filter. All I could do was stammer "Uh! Uh! Uh!" as I followed her out of the pen with my arm still stuck in her rear end (yes, that's part of the job, and yes, I wear gloves). Fortunately, the person holding the collection filter had the foresight to detach it from the tubing. We had been outsmarted by a cow.

Beef cows are just a little dumber than dairy cows. I say that affectionately since I do enjoy working with beef cattle, but what they lack in intelligence they gain in instinct. They're less domesticated, if you will. Beef cattle, almost without exception, have to be handled in a sturdy capture chute. Most of these chutes work on the premise that cows will keep moving forward as long as they see an avenue of escape. Some chutes are coupled with an automatic catch mechanism, two heavy gates that close on the cow's neck when she ties to walk through it. It's just tight enough to prevent her from backing her head out. Here's how it works: As the cow walks forward toward the locking head gate, she sees an opening just big enough for her head to fit through. As soon as her head goes through, however, she sees nothing but wide-open space and makes a break for it. When she does, her shoulders close the gate and it latches shut, restraining the cow. But some cows will balk at the gate. If the lighting is just right, and there are no other distractions, we can sometimes simply open the gate an extra inch, while the cow is watching, and she will hit the gate like a freight train. That extra inch makes it irresistible to the cow's flight instinct.

But there are also manual capture gates that require an operator to actively close the gate as the cow pokes her head through. The operator must be quick because as soon as the cow sees daylight, in the blink of an eye she could be gone. As she approaches the head gate, she walks cautiously. Already on edge, the chute operator is ready to slam the lever on his victim. The cow walks to the opening and pokes her nose through, pauses for a moment, and then suddenly . . . lowers her head to the ground.

This nifty little trick fools the chute person into slamming the gate before the cow's head is in. Realizing it's a trap, the cow balks, refusing to take another step forward. So the chute person does the only thing he can: He opens the gate a little wider. Still, the cow balks, and then, without warning, she bolts like greased lightning, escaping the clutches of the chute master.

A chute operator who has been outsmarted by a cow has to endure merciless ribbing. And a cow who has passed Chute Avoidance 101 will be even harder to catch the next time.

DELVING INTO THE PARTISAN DIVIDE

Our veterinary practice only works on food animals, and the vast majority of them are dairy cows. It's not that we don't like beef cows; on the contrary, I thoroughly enjoy working with beef cattle. It's just that they require a lot less maintenance than dairy cows and they need our assistance far less often. In fact, I sometimes marvel at the fact that beef and dairy cows are of the same species.

The contrast between beef and dairy animals is striking. The dairy cow is docile. She's been selected for this trait since man first started developing dairy breeds. It only makes sense. Her udder is right by her hind legs. If she's not the docile type, the farmer might get a swift kick in the head, which would likely hasten the cow's career to change from dairy to hamburger.

The beef cow, on the other hand, is not so docile. This makes sense too, if you consider the purpose of a beef cow is to raise a beef calf. She does this outside, in the pasture, among the coyotes and, in some parts of the country, even the wolves. A docile cow out fending for herself won't protect her mooing bundle of joy with the same zeal as one with a smidge of fire in her belly. A mama cow with just a little attitude is a good thing.

A dairy cow's frame structure differs substantially from a beef cow. The dairy cow has been developed to be tall, slightly lean, and with a deep belly so she can eat a lot. Milk production takes metabolic effort. Remember earlier when I said that a dairy cow, in peak lactation, requires as many calories for milk production as a marathon runner does to run two marathons? This is where the rubber hits the road. Or maybe where the hooves hit the dirt. The difference is that she burns that many calories every day. And don't confuse a deep belly with obesity; we want to be able to see at least a few ribs on the dairy cow. An overweight, out-of-shape cow just couldn't handle the demands of lactation.

The beef cow is a little shorter, a little rounder, and a little thicker. This comes in handy when producing a rump roast or a rib-eye steak. And it's not that milk production isn't important to a beef cow; in fact, adequate milk is imperative to raise a nice calf before weaning. But she doesn't have to run a couple of marathons every day. It's more like a 5K every now and then.

The beef calf is raised to *finish,* meaning that, when they're done growing, they deposit fat in their muscles which causes the meat to resemble marble. This fat is responsible for much of the flavor and tenderness of a nice finished beef.

Dairy breeds will also finish, many times just as nicely as a beef breed. The difference is the time it takes to finish. A beef steer can finish in as little as sixteen months, but a dairy breed may take up to two years. That's a lot of extra time and expense required for a farmer to feed and raise him.

Working a herd of beef cattle requires a good method of restraint. Beef farms typically have a very functional, strong chute system that loads cattle quickly and holds them in place once they are restrained. The cows are not at all in the mood to be there, so they quickly move through the chute in the hope that escape is possible. Just as the cow puts her head through the end of the chute, the head catch closes and temporarily restrains her. The cows are so distracted by the head lock that they barely notice me reaching up their back side to feel for the presence of a calf or the needle delivering the vaccine that will prevent disease.

Dairy cows, on the other hand, stand in a stall, sometimes unrestrained, and peacefully let me conduct the examination. Often, no chute or head catch is necessary.

The beef cow, as we try to load her into a chute, will run like she was being chased by a lion. The dairy cow rarely picks up the pace beyond a slow walk. In fact, it can be difficult to get them to move at all.

The beef cow acts like she drank too much coffee. The dairy cow acts like she hasn't a care in the world. She'll will walk up to you in the pasture and get a good sniff. Sometimes, if she's extra tame, she'll rub her head against you, wanting a good scratch in return. A dairy cow can become quite the pest.

A beef cow has two goals when they see a human in their domain. First, chase the people away so they don't try to eat her calf. Second, run away and avoid being eaten herself. The dairy cow has just *one* goal when a person enters her domain: investigate.

A dairy cow is perhaps the most fragile fifteen hundred-pound animal on the face of the Earth. If her feet aren't trimmed regularly, she just might come up lame. If her udder hair isn't clipped, she just might get an infection. If you look at her cross-eyed, she just might come down with a case of the blues. She can be high maintenance.

The beef cow has a tough streak that might impress even a Navy SEAL. I've seen severe lacerations and other injuries that would make a dairy cow give up all hope. I wouldn't give up on an injured beef cow until her heart squeezes out its last beat, and the reason is the same as her temperament. If she's out on the range and feeling a bit under the weather, the predators will pick her out as the easiest meal in the herd. Stoicism ensures that she doesn't draw attention from the wrong crowd.

Beef cows love to be outside no matter what the weather holds. They'll simply find some kind of wind break and hunker down during a storm. Dairy cows will wait by the barn door and bawl to be let back in.

Beef and dairy cows may be of the same species, but they are totally different critters. Temperament is less influenced by breed, in my opinion, than the way the animal is raised. Beef calves spend their first six months with Mama. Dairy calves, on the other hand, are hand-raised by the farmer.

When a dairy calf is raised by a beef cow, she begins to think like a beef cow. This happens when a beef cow is used as a *surrogate*, or a recipient for a dairy embryo. The beef cow raises the calf as she would her own. These beef-raised dairy calves can be remarkably wild and difficult to break. But when an orphaned beef calf is hand-raised by the farmer, it usually becomes quite tame, like a dairy calf.

Of course, these are generalizations and they do not hold true in all instances. To confuse the issue, some breeds have a dual purpose, not quite dairy cattle, and not quite beef. These are the Brown Swiss, the Milking Shorthorn, the Braunveigh, the Pinzgauer, and the Simmental, among others. Think of them as the anti-establishment breeds that don't like to be pigeonholed into dichotomous groups.

Over time, though, the dual-purpose breeds have evolved. The Brown Swiss and Milking Shorthorn are known more for their dairy ability; the Pinzgauer and Simmental are better at being beef cows, but they all still maintain some attributes of the other side.

And, to confuse the issue even more, some farmers will crossbreed beef and dairy breeds. Beef farmers might want to add some dairy influence to get a little more milk production in their beef cows. Conversely, dairy farmers might want to add some beef value to the offspring of their dairy cows. Diversity adds flexibility. The market conditions and infrastructure of each farm determine whether docile, lean dairy cows or thick, tough beef cows with attitude live there. It's as simple as that.

Right.

Regardless, the wide, wide world of cows is filled with more diversity than most people realize, and I enjoy them all the same.

COWS GET HUNGRY

I love to watch cows eat. Maybe it's because a cow's feed intake is directly proportional to her milk production. Maybe it's because feeding behavior is a microcosm of cow behavior in general. Maybe it's because I'm a little weird. Or maybe it's a combination of all three.

But if I ever have a few minutes to spare on a dairy, I make my way to the feed bunk, unfold a lawn chair, put my feet up, and watch the cows are do what cows do best—converting plant material into meat and milk.

Cows are *allelomimetic*; they all do the same thing at the same time. They like to follow the crowd. When one eats, they all eat. When one lays down, they all lay down. They're herd animals, after all.

So when fresh feed is put out for the herd, the feed bunk is where the action is. And when space is at a premium, cows protect their territory. A cow will eat with her herd mates on either side of her. If one gets too close, BAM! She lets her neighbor have it with a whack from the top of her head. Despite this threat, a cow will continue to encroach on her neighbor's territory. With a sly motion, she carefully and slowly sneaks her tongue toward the pile of feed beside her. Her neighbor's feed must taste better. Once there, a couple quick licks will steal a bite. One can almost see her grin, like she knows she's gotten away with something. In fact, cows fit into several categories based upon their chowtime habits:

- **The Sorter.** This type is well known by dairy farmers. After taking a big bite, she systematically mouths the feed and spits out the ingredients she doesn't enjoy, like my daughter used to do with lima beans. The sorter is at risk for getting sick since she doesn't eat the healthy food, only the desert.

- **The Linguist.** Perhaps the most entertaining to watch, this cow acts like she's eating an ice cream cone. She'll stick out her prehensile tongue as far as she can and sweep the manger clean of all feed. Once all the crumbs are accounted for, she will quit and chew her cud.

- **The Thief.** Also known as *greedy,* she isn't satisfied with her own portion; she has to eat her neighbor's feed too. Only after she can't reach any further to the right or left will she go to work on her own helping.

- **The Boss**. This name doesn't imply a favorite genre of music; instead it describes a personality. This cow isn't content to just reach for her neighbor's portion, she has to chase away her neighbors and any other cows that come close. Once alone, the feed is all hers.

- **The Quarterback.** This cow would make Terry Bradshaw jealous with her ability to throw a ball of feed. She takes a big bite and, without warning, chucks the feed over her back. Once a farmer knows that a cow fits this personality type, she is easy to find in the barn. Just stand at one end of the bunk and look for the feed fountain.

- Finally, there's **The Steam Shovel.** This is the cow that every farmer wants. She stands at the bunk, minds her own business, and shovels the feed without any fuss. They say the best cow in the barn is the cow that the farmer never notices, and the steam shovel fits that description.

Dairy cow rations are typically blended mixtures of several different ingredients like hay, silage, grain, and minerals. Like *The Sorter,* above, many cows will dig through the feed to find their favorite bits. If she has a taste for grain but doesn't like the forage, she will get an upset stomach, just like a child eating too much candy and not enough supper. But if a cow eats too much forage and ignores the grain, she won't consume enough calories to support her milk production. This can make her sick too. To reduce sorting, farmers take measures like maintaining proper particle size in the ration and ensuring it has enough moisture to make sorting difficult. But the cows still try.

Some dairy rations contain by-product waste like citrus pulp, beet pulp, or even expired produce from the grocery store. Cows are very green critters, especially the brown ones, the red ones, and the black-and-white ones. Cows eat stuff that would otherwise end up in the landfill. And they are happy to do their part.

I once watched a group of cows eating leftover fruits and vegetables from the local grocer. One cow was trying to sort out a spud from the pile, but she could barely reach it. She stuck out her tongue as far as she could reach and made a swipe. She missed. She pressed forward and extended her tongue again. She missed a second time. Finally, she lunged and, *bingo*, she landed it. Cows dig spuds. Not literally; that would require opposable thumbs. But they love them. The one-pound tuber disappeared into her mouth and she took a few seconds to chew it. I was glad to see that she chewed her food. If she had swallowed it whole I would probably have had to fish it out of her gullet later because a whole spud is sometimes too big to pass into the stomach. That's the sort of thing that gets the attention of a large-animal vet.

If the cows are grazing in the pasture, their idiosyncrasies change a little. Grazing behavior is essentially the same across all breeds and populations of cows. A grazing cow will extend her tongue, wrap a bunch of grass, retract her tongue and swallow. She doesn't bother to chew while she's eating; that can be don't later. Like dogs, cows treat mealtime with a high degree of urgency. She can't waste any time before her next bite.

Once she approaches the fence, she notices the grass is better on the other side. Unless the fence is electric, and even sometimes when it is, she will try to steal some of that forbidden grass. Eventually, she learns the lesson that even though the grass is greener on the other side, it isn't worth the price of an electric shock. It's a great metaphor, but I doubt that cows can grasp the rich meaning and subtlety. But we can. We can learn a lot from watching cows eat.

THE WONDER OF RUMEN

Of the cow's many awesome characteristics, *rumen* is the most awesome of all. I know what you're thinking: *Seriously?* Without a doubt. Here's why I'm a rumen enthusiast . . .

The cow belongs to a select group of animals known as ruminants which have, if you haven't already figured it out, a *rumen,* the large fermentation chamber of her complex stomach. Many people think that cows have four stomachs. Technically, they really only have one, but it has four chambers.

But she does, actually, have *fore-stomachs*. That's not a typo; they're called "fore-stomachs" because they come before the true stomach and the rumen is the largest and most interesting of these. This is where the magic happens: the conversion of indigestible forage to digestible nutrients.

Inside the rumen, trillions of bacteria, fungi, and yeast work harmoniously to break down the complex molecules of the plant matter. But the rumen is more than just a fermentation vat; a simple plastic bucket could do the same thing. The rumen constantly churns. Over and over, the rumen mixes the various layers of ingesta within its confines. It continuously mixes the liquid portion back with the solid, fibrous layers.

This fermentation produces a lot of one particular byproduct: gas. As the rumen mixes the solid with the liquid, the rumen's contractions also push the accumulating gas toward the esophagus. About every thirty seconds or so, the cow releases a hearty burp. She doesn't mean to be tactless, but unless she expels the gas, she will bloat like a balloon and die (no kidding; see Part Three for more).

In addition to the gas, the microbes produce compounds called *volatile fatty acids* from the plant material. These volatile fatty acids, unlike the bubbles of gas, are essential for the cow. *Acetic, proprionic,* and *butyric* acids are the predominant volatile fatty acids produced and the cow uses them for energy or to make milk.

As if it wasn't cool enough already, there's yet another element that makes this process even more interesting. Imagine a blade of grass that a cow just ate. A blade of grass might not be very big, but compared to the bacteria that are about to deconstruct it, it is huge. Left alone, the fermentation of a blade of grass would be a daunting task to the microbes, and the hard-working cow just doesn't have that much time.

So, after swallowing the blade of grass, the cow will chew it. You might think that the cow has it all wrong; she should chew her food *before* swallowing it. But cows like to eat on the run. She eats quickly, then finds a place to relax and chew her cud. She regurgitates a healthy portion and works on it for a while. That blade of grass becomes chewed, literally, to a pulp. This allows rumen microbes better access into the plant cells to digest it for the cow.

The rumen microbes reproduce and expand their numbers constantly, but they don't stay in the rumen indefinitely. Eventually, her other fore-stomachs allow some stuff to pass through. As the feed particles are spent and leave the rumen, a stream of microbes follows. These microbes are, in turn, digested by the cow in a more traditional manner, providing the cow with a lot of protein, among other important nutrients.

As you might imagine, this fermentation is a delicately balanced process. If any one thing gets out of whack, as might happen after a drastic feed change for example, the cow can get a nasty case of indigestion, or worse. Disorders of the rumen, like bloat or acute acidosis, can kill a cow.

But hundreds of millions of bovines worldwide, each of them with trillions of microbes in their rumens, convert plant material into protein. Plant material that is indigestible to humans becomes edible meat or dairy products. It's nothing short of a miracle.

FARTS:
SO MUCH MORE THAN ADOLESCENT HUMOR

Cows are allegedly destroying the planet with their flatulence. They do tend to be gassy, but all kidding aside, the theory goes like this: Cows eat forage. A byproduct of forage digestion is *methane*. This gas is released in an unfiltered tailwind directly into the atmosphere. Since methane is a much more potent greenhouse gas than carbon dioxide is, it could have the potential to cause environmental harm.

We know that cows produce methane during the fermentative digestion of their feed, and they can be prolific gas producers, on the order of a liter or so a minute. Most of the produced methane is actually belched (cows burp about twice a minute), but cow flatulence is much more interesting to discuss, and only slightly less polite.

There must be a solution to this crisis. We could get rid of cows . . . Just kidding, that's not an option. But it has been suggested by some, even some in our own government. It's about as popular with my people as a barking spider in church.

We could stuff a cork in the cows to prevent the release of air biscuits. On second thought, that would ruin a cow's day in short order. Remember bloat? If a cow gets an obstruction at either end of the digestive tract, the gas has nowhere to go and accumulates. If the obstruction is toward the rear, she becomes uncomfortable and her girth expands a little. But if the obstruction is near the front, preventing her from burping, it can be quickly fatal. The accumulating gas expands the cow like an inelastic balloon. All that pressure on her insides causes major problems, like inability to breathe and total circulatory collapse. So let's not suggest stuffing cows with corks.

We could insert an ignition system to burn off the methane as the cows backfire. Try to imagine the nation's barnyards lit up like an oil refinery at night. Beautiful. Here's the problem: Barns contain cows and flammable hay. Flaming cows and dry hay are a sure-fire recipe for a real barn burner.

So are there any good options for the harm that the unwitting cow is doing to our environment? First of all, I sincerely wish that some people would stop scapegoating the cow. Please, leave the poor cow alone; she means no harm. After all, there are nearly a billion bovines worldwide with about ten percent of them living in the US. Cows are not the villains. Truth is, the environmental footprint of the cow has been steadily shrinking relative to the US human population. Modern farming methods lead to lower bovine methane production, and cattle that are fed primarily high-grain diets will produce less methane than cattle on grass or hay diets. High grain rations can also finish a beef in shorter time than one finished on grass, which also cuts the total methane produced during its lifetime. Dairy cattle fed grain in their rations produce more milk than if fed grass alone, reducing methane production per unit of milk.

Second, as farmers select for better and more efficient cows, their carbon footprint will continue to decline. Farmers and cows both continue to get better at what they do. Dairy farmers today produce more milk with fewer cows. Beef animals grow faster with better carcass characteristics than decades ago. This means more meat and milk produced from fewer animals. Fewer animals produce less methane.

Third, cow manure management is a contributor to the overall carbon footprint of cattle. Agricultural engineers and farmers have figured out a way to capture the methane produced as the manure is stored. This methane can either be burned or, better yet, used as fuel for a methane-powered electric generator. There are, I believe, four of those already in my county in Pennsylvania alone.

Philosophically, what's a person who cares about the environment to do? We have to eat, after all. Agricultural activities in 2017, according to the EPA, accounted for only 8.4% of all greenhouse gas emissions in the US. Methane by all livestock, including cattle, were about 32% of agriculture's contribution, or roughly 2.7% of all man-made greenhouse gas production. Even if cows didn't exist, food production would still emit significant and substantial greenhouse gasses. Meatless Mondays will do nothing to save the polar ice caps. No, the solution isn't to eliminate cows. That would really stink.

THE MAJESTIC COW

Size matters. Looks are important. Cows are rarely judged by their beauty and superficial characteristics, except when they are. Some cows are in show business, and I'm not talking about Elsie. The prized show cow at the county fair is most certainly a source of pride for the farmer, but it goes deeper than that. And beauty for the cow is more than just skin deep. It goes all the way to her bones.

The entire competition is analogous to a beauty pageant. The red carpet and runway are replaced by wood chips and an arena. Evening gowns are replaced by finely groomed fur. Mingling with the contestants is allowed, but I'll warn you, you might want to wear boots and keep your eyes on the floor.

Historically, the cow show began as a means to identify the best and most profitable cows, not just the prettiest. There is a single judge, not a panel, and his word is final. The judge looks for specific characteristics: The cow has to be sound in her feet and legs since a lame cow doesn't get around very well, and she should have a big, wide frame, which allows her to deliver a calf with ease and eat a lot of feed to support her high milk production. Making milk takes a lot of calories and if she can't eat a lot, she can't milk a lot.

But she can't be fat either, and curves are a detriment. No, the pretty show cow should be angular and thin, not curvy. But most importantly, she has to have a nice udder that is attached tightly to her body. Tampering with Mother Nature is strictly forbidden too, so each winner is tested for the presence of silicone. That's no joke; it really is. Size matters here too, but simply being well-endowed isn't enough. Think of where the udder is on the cow: It's located on her belly. Gravity, over time, takes its toll. If the udder doesn't have strong attachments to the body, it can sag.

Saggy is not good if you're a cow. It's not because farmers just like to look at pretty udders, no, that would be weird. But a milking unit can't attach to an udder properly if it's too low. Looks are important, but not just for the sake of being pretty. The reality is that function follows form.

The cow show has, in some respects, taken on a life of its own. There are outward qualities of the cow that are imperative for function, like feet and legs and the udder, but there are also qualities that can't be judged from the outside. Some of the beauty of a good, profitable cow comes from within. She must be healthy and have a strong immune system. She must be able to produce milk with lots of protein and milk fat. These traits don't appear on the outside but can only be established through the test of time or genetic testing. Those tools are available to the farmer today.

Being beautiful doesn't come easy for a cow. It takes work. She has to keep herself in shape, yes, but all that hair still needs grooming. There are well-qualified people called fitters who make a living grooming cows for the show ring, sales, or even photographs (Yes, some cows get to be models). These folks are true professionals and artists without all of an artist's baggage. A spa treatment for a cow consists of a long, cool shower and a figurative shoeshine. Cows like it cool, so a garden hose is as good as a bubble bath.

Once the schmutz is removed, she gets a haircut. Most of her hair is taken down to the level of a buzz cut save one thing: the switch hair on her tail. That hair is combed and teased and combed and cleaned and teased some more until it puffs out like a big 1980s hairdo. And the best fitters will even prepare the fur on her top line to be as straight as an arrow to accentuate her angularity.

The eventual winner of the show is awarded with a blue ribbon and a small cash prize, but not enough to cover all the costs associated with preparing for and attending the show. There is also the pride of having a champion, but it doesn't end there. The real payoff can come through the sale of offspring or even of the cow herself.

The stakes can be quite high, in fact. A winner of a national show can fetch up to six figures, sometimes more. And the offspring from a contender at a national show can fetch ten times the value of a grade calf. But lest you think this is an easy way to make some quick scratch, it isn't. Being pretty is hard work.

The cow, indeed, is a majestic creature. The farmer, for his part, is the steward of her majesty. But my part as the veterinarian, well, I function behind the scenes to keep her healthy, productive, and prolific.

Part Three
COW DOCTORS MAKE HOUSE CALLS

Doctor-patient communication is an essential component of health care. So when people ask me how I know what's wrong with my patients, my reply is, "Good question!" The nonverbal nature of cows does pose a problem sometimes, but their symptoms usually give me a clue. And a good physical exam can start to point me in the right direction.

But worse than my patient's inability to communicate with me is my inability to communicate with my patient. When attempting to give an injection, it's hard to warn the patient not to kick. We can say, "Little pinch . . ." if we want to, but all the cow hears is, "Blah, blah, blah . . ." And as soon as that little pinch hits her hide her rear foot goes airborne.

Any procedure on an animal must be done with the expectation that the patient will misinterpret the intention. There are times I wish I could be the cow whisperer. Life would be easier if I could give fair warning or even instructions.

When trying to pen an animal, giving detailed, yet simple instructions just isn't an option. There are several directions from which the critter can choose, but we want her to go in only one. Instead of telling her what to do, which nobody likes, we trick her into thinking we're going to grab her. She wants to escape, but the only option we leave her is the pen that we want her to inhabit.

When delivering calves, it would be nice if we could instruct the patient to push when it's necessary and stop pushing when it's not. It's inappropriate to push when I'm in her up to my armpit trying to untangle a misdirected calf. That can cause problems. Cows can muster enough power to push a golf ball through a fifty-foot garden hose, so imagine the pressure when my hand gets stuck between the calf and her birth canal during a contraction. I always yell, "Stop pushing!" But they never listen.

And once we get the calf headed in the right direction, it would be nice to ask for a little help. "Push! Push!" is usually ignored. And when she won't listen, traction on the calf has to be supplied by the vet and the farmer.

Perhaps the most frustrating time to suffer a lack of communication is when there's an emergency. The veins that drain the udder are both enormous and superficial; it's a recipe for disaster. One nick from a barbed-wire fence can leave a cow with one foot in the grave and the other three on banana peels. Simple skin sutures in the lacerated vein are the remedy, but the udder is on the underside of the cow. It's hard enough to place sutures in a moving target, even harder when it's standing upright with the moving target on her belly. It would be nice to have the ability to impart the gravity of the situation to the victim. "Quit kicking me!" just makes her kick harder as the suture drags through her skin. Eventually, though, the sutures get placed, and hopefully without any new lumps on the surgeon's head.

A prolapsed uterus is another emergency that the cow fails to understand. This can happen immediately after the cow delivers her calf: The uterus passes through the birth canal, like removing your sweatshirt by turning it inside out, and gets trapped on the outside of the cow. This organ weighs about sixty pounds and has a tremendous blood supply. If not replaced within a couple of hours, the cow is at serious risk of death. But does she know that? Of course not.

For the veterinarian, it's much easier to replace a prolapse while the cow is prone on the ground. So I like to tell her, "Don't get up! Don't get up!" It's good advice, but she doesn't always listen. Again, what we have here is a failure to communicate.

If she gets on her feet (good luck stopping her) and her womb drapes down, we have to work against gravity. I usually have assistants support the large, swinging uterus on a smooth wooden plank. As I start to work the uterus back in place, the patient gets a little anxious and begins to swing her rear end from side to side. Again, I say "Stand still!" but she never listens.

As I make progress, the *Ferguson reflex* kicks in, which is a nearly uncontrollable urge to push when something is in the birth canal, like a calf, the vet's arm, or half a uterus. It's exactly the sort of thing that I don't want to have to deal with when I've just spent twenty minutes pushing her insides back in from the outside.

The prolapsed uterus was probably best described by James Herriot many years ago. To paraphrase, the veterinarian works and works to the point of exhaustion just to have the cow undo all of the progress in the instant just before the job is done. I have my own reflex in that situation: I yell, "ARRRRGH! Quit pushing!" to no avail. Back to the drawing board.

As a species, humans have figured out how to communicate with each other by sounds, words, pictures, hand signs, computers, text message, social media, smoke signals, and countless other ways. Maybe someday we'll find a way to talk to the cows. I wonder what they'll say in return?

COW DOCTORS AND HOW TO BE ONE

Why would anyone want to do what I do? Aside from trying to talk to the cows, I get to work with some of the finest people on the planet: American farmers. You'll never find a harder-working, more dedicated, and more loyal group of folks, and when one of them encounters hard times you can count on the others to help out. They're competitive, but they're also a big family. That's my crowd.

I also have a deep and abiding interest in animal welfare, yet I also believe in the hierarchy of species: Animals are here to serve mankind. Some see this as a contradiction. I see it as a contract. If cows provide us with meat and leather and milk and cheese, then we owe it to the cows to ensure that their lives are as healthy and comfortable as reasonably possible. And cows that are healthy and comfortable provide a better return for the farmer. It's a win-win, and my role in maintaining man's contract with the cows is an essential one.

If you want to be a large-animal vet and reap the rich barnyard rewards that the career provides, you have to commit yourself to long days in the field and continuous ongoing education and self-improvement. When I graduated from Virginia-Maryland Regional College of Veterinary Medicine, most of what I was taught and had read in the textbooks was already obsolete. Now that's not a criticism of my alma mater, but knowledge advances so quickly that the textbooks can't keep up, and sometimes it's even hard for the teachers.

Granted, that means that as technology advances, the vets also have to keep up. We never stop learning. After years in the classrooms and in the field doing practical work, the farms of America become our schools. In fact, class is in session every day that I'm on the job (which is pretty much every day).

And don't be like the law student who quit after a few months because it "isn't like it is on TV." Find out what the job is like before settling into a program of study and shelling out the dough. Since I'm in large-animal practice, I don't have much to do with companion animals and that's by design. A client will occasionally ask me to examine a litter of puppies to make sure they're all healthy, or administer a rabies shot to a working dog, but I'm otherwise pretty much all about the cows. I knew that because I had been around them, one way or another, most of my life and I had an educated idea of what spending your days with cows would be like. After a brief but failed experiment with the profession of pharmacy, I gazed across the open pastureland at the serenely grazing livestock and said, "Yep, that's for me."

I'm having a little fun with this, but the decision to enter veterinary school shouldn't be taken lightly. It's a lot of work and the cost of the education is high. Veterinary schools generally do a fine job of selecting candidates who understand the commitment that the career field requires.

As a veterinarian, I love my profession. I am reminded of how fortunate I am every time a person tells me that they have a child, niece, or nephew who wants to attend veterinary school. I feel a sense of pride every time I hear a young person say he or she wants to be a vet. While the hours can be longer and the pay shorter than other professions, it is nonetheless the most fulfilling job I can see myself doing.

I worry, though, that some who desire to enter the profession of veterinary medicine don't know what they might be getting. It's not about loving animals. If I were ever on the admissions committee for a veterinary school, I would automatically disqualify any applicant who said he or she wanted to be a veterinarian because "I love animals."

That is a provocative statement. Many people love animals including, I'm sure, a good many people reading this. I don't discount the importance that animals play in our lives, but loving animals is not an appropriate reason to want to be a veterinarian.

I am a veterinarian because I've always wanted to work with farmers, specifically farmers who raise livestock. Animals never pick up the phone to call the veterinarian; their person does. Animals never take the advice of their veterinarian; their person does. Animals never pay their veterinary bill; their person does, hopefully.

The profession of veterinary medicine is one of service, especially clinical practice. If I could advise anyone preparing to enter this field, I would suggest falling in love with the science, not the patients, and be prepared to serve. Let the challenge of solving problems and learning new things be your motivation.

There is a plethora of specialties within the profession, like ophthalmology, radiology, anesthesia, neurology, clinical pathology, theriogenology (reproduction), as well as government regulatory positions and corporate endeavors. The mainstay of the profession still is, however, private clinical practice.

And by no means should a person consider the long, expensive, grueling educational experience without an exact knowledge of the consequences. Veterinary education is more than expensive. A new car is expensive; a veterinary education is nearly cost prohibitive. It's not uncommon for debt loads of graduating veterinarians to exceed a quarter-million dollars, and starting salaries for new graduates aren't necessarily proportional to the cost of the education.

One should consider exactly what will be expected of him or her once in clinical practice, if that is the avenue of choice. Every office visit is not a new puppy check, nor is it a friendly Golden Retriever with a repairable broken bone. It might just be a fractious cat with razor sharp claws and fangs waiting to sink into the arm of the one who's trying to take a rectal temperature. Or it could be the aging best friend with a chronic disease that the clinician has treated for years who presents for euthanasia. Again, the profession is about service.

If entering large animal practice, expect to be available at any hour of the day or night to patch up a broken cow or horse, deliver a calf, or treat an ailing goat. But if a person thinks that they can take the bad along with the good, in the end there ends up being more good than bad.

I have zero regrets about the decision I made some thirty years ago, but I did walk into it with both eyes open. I am fascinated by science and I love working with farmers. I don't mind cow poop and I can tolerate miserable weather. I like animals, yes, but if that had been my primary motivation, I would have left the profession decades ago. It isn't like retail sales or office work, thank goodness. It's rough-and-tumble and if you don't know what you're getting into, you're likely to regret it.

THAT SILVER-TONGUED, HANDSOME DOCTOR . . . Which brings us back to communication. Aside from anatomy, immunology, internal medicine, and a host of other topics, communication is one of the fields that a veterinarian must master to be successful. Communicating with cows is hard (see above). Communicating with people isn't necessarily easy either. In school we were told that we could be the best and smartest clinician in the world, but if we lacked the ability to communicate effectively to the owner of the critter we were dealing with, we would fail.

The ability to communicate with farmers and, at the same time, other clinicians becomes even more interesting when one considers the vernacular used by farmers to describe disease, most of which are privy only to those who actually have a role in dealing with these animals.

Descriptions from *wooden tongue* to *heaves* sometimes adequately describe symptoms to the layperson, but the definitive description is usually reserved for us pointy-headed doctor types when we communicate amongst ourselves. It's not because we're snobs. Well, most of us aren't. The definitive medical terminology allows us to converse with colleagues without any ambiguity, but it leaves everyone else in the dark. The no-nonsense nature of farmers ensures that they have their own terminology and, while it may not be clinically correct, it sure is a heck of a lot more entertaining. See what you think.

Foot rot describes a common disease in cattle that causes lameness. Medical types such as myself have dubbed it *interdigital dermatitis* because the skin between the hooves becomes infected until it literally smells rotten. Fortunately, a shot of antibiotic usually clears it up within a day or two.

Twisted stomach is one of my all-time favorite maladies. As the name suggests, the stomach, or at least one of its chambers, twists and gets trapped in the wrong position. Doctors like to call this one *displaced abomasum* and, fortunately again for the cow, this one is usually repairable with surgery.

Lumpy jaw. If you've ever seen a cow with this disease, you'd appreciate its name. The cow's jaw literally develops a big lump on it, a much bigger one that you would expect to see on a cow that's simply saving a cud for a later chew. *Actinomycosis*, as we veterinarians like to call it, is caused by a bacterial infection that gets into the jawbone and, if treated early, it can be cured with surgery. But it's an expensive fix that is only attempted on the most valuable cows.

Circling disease. If you inferred by the name that the affected animal walks around in circles, you'd be right. Veterinarians call this one *Listeriosis* because it's caused by a *Listeria* bacterium which infects the nerves in the ear and the brain that help maintain balance. These poor animals can also make a full recovery if treated early.

Cancer eye. The scientific name for this one is a real mouthful—*ocular squamous cell carcinoma*—and it really is a cancer of the cow's eye. It's the only cancer that we ever attempt to treat in a cow because it can be cured if we remove all of the cancer before it has spread. Sometimes this means that we have to take the whole eye.

Fortunately for the cow, the Good Lord gave her a spare just in case.

Cockarosis. Most people haven't heard of this one. One morning our receptionist informed me that a farmer had called to say that his calf had the cockarosis. I said, "*What?*" Being a recently graduated veterinarian, I figured it was just the local vernacular for some interesting disease so I signed up for the call. This farmer was the rough, hard-working type and he always sported a big chew of tobacco. Sometimes he bit off more than he could chew and it had the tendency to affect his speech. When I arrived on his farm and asked him what he thought was ailing the calf, he told me that she had the cockarosis. I said, "*What?*" He had to repeat himself several times before he finally revealed that the calf had diarrhea. It was only then that I figured out that she had a case of *coccidiosis* which commonly affects calves and gives them a nasty bout of diarrhea. It is easily treated with medicine to kill the offending parasite, but only if you can decipher the farmer's tobacco-impaired speech.

Hollow tail might be my favorite, describing the condition of a cow that is down in the pasture and can't get up. I've actually never seen a case in Pennsylvania, but it was common in rural southwest Virginia where I went to veterinary school. At least it was *thought* to be common. The medical consensus is that it probably happens only after a Chupacabra attack. As you might have already guessed, there is no scientific name for this one.

. . . AND THOSE TONGUE-TIED COWS

Even if cows could talk they still might not tell us what's wrong. Biologists tell us that prey species, like cows, hide sickness so they won't tempt predators and become an easy meal. A cow that looks sick is likely to get eaten by the wolfpack.

I've done many post-mortem exams that left me scratching my head, not because I was confused but because of the extent of the pathology. Sometimes the disease is so severe, it's amazing the animal survived as long as it did. This points to another characteristic of cows: They're tough. Masking sickness in order to stay alive requires incredible stamina and endurance, not to mention acting ability. How many of us could go about our daily business, with no changes in our behavior, while hiding a painful, agonizing condition? I'm pretty tough, but I have my limits. I don't think I could do it. Cows do it all the time.

Sometimes something beyond the cow's control gives away the presence of a condition. It could be a change in milk production, telltale signs in the fecal matter, or any number of other things. When this happens, veterinarians attempt to figure out what's wrong and prognosticate the likelihood of both survival and return to production. In the case of cows in need of abdominal surgery to fix a twisted-up gut, we use several parameters to predict outcome. Heart rate is one of the best indicators. A heart rate of 100 to 120 beats per minute indicates severe pain and distress and arguably carries a poor prognosis for survival.

The cow's attitude and how she holds her ears can also give some clues to the prognosis, as do the appearance of the cow's eyes. Depressed attitude and droopy ears are bad signs. If the eyeballs are sunken into their sockets the cow may suffer from significant dehydration. If the whites of the eyes appear bloodshot, or injected, there may be a blood infection.

When a cow's stomach twists to the left, it is a pretty easy fix surgically and it carries a good prognosis. But if the stomach twists to the right, the blood supply to the stomach can be disrupted and the prognosis is always guarded. We use heart rate and appearance of the eyes to predict the degree of severity of a right-twisted stomach in the patient, but it isn't a perfect prognostic tool and sometimes we get fooled.

I was called by a farmer once for a dairy cow that had a right-side twisted stomach. I did my usual pre-surgery assessment and the cow looked like an excellent candidate for surgery. Her heart rate was only slightly elevated and her eyes looked fine. I even remarked to the farmer that I felt the cow must have just gotten sick. He agreed.

When I opened her abdomen, I was greeted with a terrible sight and smell. Her stomach had ruptured and she was filled with infection. It was not a recent injury and I would never have guessed the severity of her condition. She had likely been walking around with this going on inside of her for a few days. *Tough.* Sadly, we had no choice but to euthanize her.

When it comes to toughness, the beef cow is in a class by itself. A beef cow is quite capable of delivering a calf, cleaning it off for thirty minutes or so, and then watching the baby calf stand upright and walk alongside of her. That feat, in and of itself, indicates toughness. Sometimes, though, things don't go as planned.

If the calf isn't positioned correctly at the time of birth, the cow can't deliver it. Beef cows, being the stoic type, will tolerate the pain and behave as if everything is hunky-dory. That is, until the calf dies and begins to decompose. We've all enjoyed the experience of the roadkill groundhog that's been allowed to ferment for three days in the summer sun, so I don't need to describe the aroma. Unfortunately, the same rankness emanates from inside the cow when its calf dies in utero. I get to help these cows occasionally, and one in particular sticks in my mind. She never let on that there was a problem, but every predator within two miles downwind already knew. I'll spare you the details, but after delivering the stillborn calf I smelled worse than the cow. Then she stood and walked away as if nothing had ever been wrong. *Tough.*

IT'S A TOUGH PILL TO SWALLOW

There's that word again: *tough.* One thing about being a veterinarian: Some of the things we deal with aren't pretty, and they don't smell good either. I wanted to get a few of the worst-case scenarios out of the way early to toughen up my readers (see what I did there?). Sometimes we get lucky and can treat a condition just by asking a cow to swallow a pill. Sadly, it's rarely that simple.

Cows don't like to take pills. To pill a dog, try rewarding him with a treat. If your dog isn't especially trainable, hide the pill in a lump of peanut butter and he'll eat it right up. Finicky dogs will scour off the peanut butter and deposit the sparkling-clean pill on the floor, uneaten. Thankfully, not many dogs are finicky. Most will eat anything, but if yours gives you a hard time, try wrapping the pill in a piece of cheese. Cheese is smellier. If all of these fail you can always resort to the drastic measure of gaping his jaws open and pushing the pill down the old gullet with your index finger. Pill taken; mission accomplished.

Cats, on the other hand, are uncooperative by nature and never fall for these tricks. Brute force is the only thing that works. A quick but firm sneak attack to push the pill down its throat is sometimes effective by the fourth or fifth attempt, but be sure to wear a leather jacket because your beloved pet is likely to retaliate with some therapeutic bloodletting.

Cows don't like pills either. The cow has about a half-ton advantage on the farmer, so some heavy-duty restraint is imperative (although it should be noted that cows, unlike cats, do not have sharp claws). There is even a metal tool used to pill a cow since trying to push the pill down her throat with your hand would likely leave you with a bloody stump where your finger used to be.

Fortunately, I don't have to pill cows very often. There just aren't that many options to treat a cow with oral medicine because the cows have what dogs and cats (and people) do not—a rumen, the large fermentation chamber of the complex forestomach that makes a ruminant a ruminant. The normal microbial flora of the rumen tends to break down many of the drugs that could be used, or at least dilute them to the point that they're ineffective.

But there are exceptions. Sometimes you can give a cow an aspirin, or *twenty* aspirins, but oral medicines usually act either directly on the rumen or use the rumen to make them effective, turning the organ into part of the treatment process, and the medications aren't always in pill form.

Here's an example: Beer has been used as an oral remedy for cows that are off their feed, or won't eat. How does it work? Well, I don't think anyone knows for sure, but people smarter than I am say it supplies some of the fermentation byproducts that an off-feed cow lacks. Beer is a fermented drink, after all. Or maybe it just gives her the drunken munchies.

There was a time when most dairy barns were stocked with a couple twelve-packs of Pabst. After wrestling with a finicky cow to administer a couple cans of beer, the farmer might be inclined to kick back a cold one himself. At least it would make the *farmer* feel better. Whiskey is used for only the most stubborn cases.

Then there's the case of the bloat. Cows can develop a severely distended rumen caused by rapid gas accumulation. The fermentation process can produce a liter of gas every minute. If the cow can't burp the gas stays put and builds up pressure. Think of the last time you ate too much chili and multiply it by ten.

Bloat can also be caused by an accumulation of foam that prevents the cow from burping, just like the suds on the beer the farmer just gave her. But this foam won't disperse without help. A common remedy is to drench the bloated cow's rumen with a mixture of one-part vegetable oil, one-part liquid soap, and six-parts water—in other words, an oily bubble bath.

Just to avoid any misunderstanding, the word *drench* used in the context of treating a cow means to administer the liquid medication orally. I usually prescribe an Epsom salt drench as a supplement for a cow suffering from magnesium deficiency. Epsom salts are perhaps the best oral treatment for magnesium deficiency, also called *grass tetany* or *hypomagnesemia*, as the vets call it. One farmer took it out of context and, after a few days, asked how long he should drench the cow's back with the dissolved Epsom salts. Fortunately for the cow, she had already responded to the intravenous treatment I had given her and was doing fine, but a little soggy. Anyways . . .

Getting back to the oily bubble bath, I know it seems counterintuitive to use soap to dissolve suds, but the oil makes it an effective *surfactant* which breaks down the stubborn foam in the rumen. It's important to keep the cow away from open flames once she starts burping again, otherwise the neighbors might think there's a new gas well next door.

There are other interesting home remedies farmers can use to treat cows orally, some of them effective, some epic failures. All of the homeopathic remedies fall into the latter category, but they do at least supply one necessary substance: water.

I learned about another epic fail in veterinary school. The inside of the rumen needs some *scratch*. This isn't the scratch you give to a dog behind his ear; no, it's more of a constant, can't-live-without-it type of scratch. This scratch is typically long-stem plant fiber that stimulates movement and fermentation by gently scratching the inside surfaces of the rumen. The problem with this situation is that long-stem plant fiber isn't very digestible and, as necessary as it is, it mostly just takes up space. Some researchers thought, *If we can replace that long stem fiber with something a little more permanent, something that doesn't occupy so much of the rumen's space, we could feed the cows more good stuff and they will be more productive.* So they tried long-stem plastic.

In theory, the plastic would provide the necessary scratch for the rumen to be stimulated. In practice, the cows regurgitated the plastic, chewed it to a fine plastic pulp right along with their cud, and you know the rest of the story. I don't think the study ever got published.

The rumen complicates our ability to treat a cow orally (as if it wasn't already complicated enough), but at least they're easier to treat than cats.

FROM MOUTH TO TAIL

There are some procedures, such as dehorning, castration, and the much-maligned tail docking that, at first glance, may seem unnecessary and stressful. They are also painful; I don't dispute that. Fortunately, there is ongoing research into pain mitigation and there's no doubt that much more will be done in the future. But while these procedures may seem unnecessary, or even purely cosmetic, to those who don't hang out with cows, there are legitimate reasons to perform them.

Horns are an obvious problem among herd animals, potentially allowing them to cause tremendous injuries to one another (not to mention the farmer and the vet). It's better to take a preemptive approach and do away with the horns entirely than it is to treat the horrific and even life-threatening gashes that could occur if they're allowed to grow.

Castration helps prevent fighting among bulls and to prevent pregnancy in female animals being fed for beef (pregnancy in the barnyard is managed and controlled by the farmer). A mature bull is aggressive toward other animals and people. A pen full of bulls is even worse.

A castrated bull is called a *steer* and, in addition to the improved behavioral disposition of steers, there are meat-quality issues that lend credence to the practice of castrating bulls before they reach puberty. Many believe, and I am in this camp, that steers make a better finished beef than bulls. The end product, remember, is *beef*, not just hamburger. Premium cuts, like steaks and roasts, must be the best that they can be if farmers want to continue to have a market.

But what of tail docking? Is this necessary, or should the practice be outlawed? This is far from a cut-and-dried issue. Some states have outlawed tail removal; in states where it's still allowed, many milk processors have prohibited the practice for the farms that supply their milk.

The question, though, is why some farmers want to remove the tails of their cows in the first place. First, consider the ultimate purpose of a cow's tail: It's to swat the flies that buzz around her top line. When the flies bother her, she gives a good whack with her tail and they scatter. If you watch a cow grazing in the summer, you'll see that her tail swishes almost non-stop.

But the tail is at, well, the tail-end of the cow. At the tip of the tail is some very long and thick hair called the *switch*. And you know what else comes out the tail end of the cow. The switch becomes a manure trap and, over time, may resemble some unspeakable torture device from the Spanish Inquisition.

Once the switch becomes caked with effluent from the cow's rear, she can use it to fling wet poo from one end of the barn to the other. She'll paint her own body with it from her top line to her udder. Early in the history of tail docking, there was evidence that removing a cow's tail improved cleanliness in cows housed in dairy barns, and this cleanliness could potentially result in less udder infections, making tailless cows *healthier* cows.

Since then, though, it's been difficult to prove scientifically that docking tails reduces the incidence of udder infections (called *mastitis*). Nonetheless, cows without tails do remain cleaner. And I can guarantee that a cow with a docked tail will never smack a farmer or his vet in the face with a dirty tail.

That being said, does it justify the practice of removing the tails of cows? I believe it could. If the primary function of the tail is fly control on pasture, does the dairy cow really need a tail? After all, dairy cattle are mostly housed in barns ventilated in a way that controls swarms of flies. Flies can also be controlled, to a degree, with pesticides and parasitic wasps. A dairy cow without a tail will never really miss it.

How are tails removed? Typically, this is done before the cow has her first calf, and almost always done by applying a strong rubber band at about one third the length of the tail from where it attaches to the body. This constricts the blood flow, depriving the tail of sensation (just like how your arm can "go to sleep" if you lay on it funny). Then the tail beyond the rubber band dies and sloughs after a week or so. With a little local anesthesia applied through an epidural injection, it can be a painless procedure.

Even so, the practice is controversial among dairy farmers, some swearing they would never consider removing a tail unless it was injured beyond repair. And animal rights activists have called the practice barbaric and used the issue as a blunt tool with which to figuratively beat dairy farmers over the head.

Routine practices such as dehorning, castration, and tail docking have proven useful for farmers for the long-term health benefits in the herds of cattle which they oversee. They cost the farmer time and money to perform and are not merely surgeries of convenience (if they were, they wouldn't do them). They have benefits for the animals, the people who work with them, and the food they produce. Castration and dehorning have become time-tested, accepted husbandry procedures. Unfortunately, the picture depicting the "barbaric" practice of tail docking was, I believe, painted with a dirty switch.

ANIMAL MAGNETISM

I have no idea how magnets work. I understand the theory: There's a north pole and a south pole. The north pole repels another north pole but attracts the south pole and vice versa. I understand the theory, but I don't know how they work. The underlying mechanics are a mystery to me.

But work they do, and it's a good thing. Magnetic force is responsible for much of our electric power generation. Without it, there would be no electric light, no alternator to recharge your car battery, no electric water heaters, and no rechargeable laptop computer from which

I could write this book. In fact, there's a magnet inside my computer. I still don't know how it works.

Cows don't know how they work either, and I doubt they know much about the theory. But human beings know that magnets attract steel, a little factoid that has tremendous implications for the well-being of cows. Here's why: Cows are indiscriminate eaters. They plow through their grub like a machine, swallowing everything they can as fast as they can. If there's a nail or a wire lost in the grass or feed bunk, it will probably get swallowed by a cow. Other species are significantly more careful about what they eat, but cows are all about quantity over quality. Whatever fills their bellies is just fine.

But what about that stray nail or wire that just shot down the cow's throat? The cow's complex forestomach is responsible for mixing and sorting the feed after she's already eaten it. Once the swallowed particles are small enough, often after having been rechewed two or three times, they are allowed to pass down the line for further digestion. Larger plant material gets held back for further regurgitation and cud-chewing.

Foreign objects like nails and wires are heavier than the plant material and they sink to the reticulum, the lowest part of the first chamber of the stomach. The reticulum is essentially a muscular bag with three opening that sort the cow's feed: some of it remains in the largest chamber (the rumen) for fermentation, some is regurgitated for further processing (chewing), and some is passed down the line for digestion. Wires, nails, and other heavy indigestible objects sink to the bottom of the reticulum and are likely to stay there. A sharp wire or nail might puncture the reticulum, and a punctured reticulum will ruin a cow's day. Farmers call this *hardware disease,* veterinarians call it *traumatic reticuloperitonitis.*

Anatomically, the reticulum lies is a precarious position within the cow's belly, immediately behind the heart. A nail or wire popping through the reticulum could puncture the heart as well, a nearly always fatal injury. On the brighter side, it could just penetrate into the body cavity causing only a nasty, life-threatening infection and digestive dysfunction.

Here's where the magnet saves the day. If a farmer forces a cow to swallow a magnet, it will also find its way to the reticulum and attract the offending object, rendering it unable to puncture anything. It'll just churn around harmlessly in the reticulum for the life of the cow.

This is no ordinary magnet, though. It's a really big and strong magnet, the kind that could entertain your kids for hours. It's not as big and strong as the ones used in junk yards to lift cars. That would be overkill. But it's still bigger than the ones that hold the juvenile art gallery to your refrigerator door. This magnet is about the size of a generous breakfast sausage link. And it's powerful. It's powerful enough to make separating two hardware magnets a difficult chore.

How do you get a cow to swallow a magnet? The farmer—or the vet—stuffs it down the cow's throat by using a tool meant for dosing cows with large pills called a balling gun. From there, it finds its own way to the bottom of the reticulum. Some farmers do this when they suspect a cow has hardware disease, but many do it preventatively, feeding a magnet as soon as she's big enough to swallow it.

How do you know if your cow has a magnet? Use a compass. *Fascinating.*

HOLEY COW

Usually, when a cow has a hole in it, it's my job to close it up. Why on earth would I want to create one unless it's for surgery (in which case I would *still* be closing it up)? Easy. A *fistulated* cow is a cow with a permanent, surgically created hole in her side that extends into the rumen. The surgery is relatively easy to perform and there is even a commercially available insert that can be placed around the fistula to prevent its natural closure. It comes with a handy lid to prevent the leakage of the stinky rumen contents.

Okay, but why would a vet want to do such a bizarre thing? First, it makes an ideal teaching tool for veterinary and animal science students. It allows for direct observation of the inside of the forestomach of a cow. When I was in veterinary school, we were taught to reach inside the fistula, locate the reticulum, and find the magnet. Once your arm is inside the rumen of a live cow, the internal anatomy can be felt and appreciated. And the aroma is not to be missed.

Another reason is strictly for research purposes. In order to determine the digestibility of certain diets, feed is placed in a permeable bag and left inside the fistulated rumen of a cow for forty-eight hours. Then the bag is removed and the contents are analyzed. The difference between what went in and what came out is the part that was digested by the rumen microorganisms. One of the best uses for a fistulated cow is to provide nutritional support for sick cows. When a cow gets sick, the rumen may quit functioning correctly and the microorganisms normally populating the rumen that are responsible for the fermentation process will die off. If a farm has access to a fistulated cow, they can harvest "rumen juice," containing millions and millions of normal bacteria and other single-celled organisms and transfer it to the sick cow by pumping it through a stomach tube. If successful, the sick cow's rumen is repopulated with normal, healthy microorganisms and she starts to eat again. It's the only practical transplant procedure done in cows.

A farm without a fistulated cow can also experience the benefit of some rumen juice if it can be borrowed from another farm that does have one. The transplant, however, must be done quickly. If the juice is left alone for more than a few hours, the population of bacteria will change, rendering it useless. And since the microorganisms are actively fermenting, they produce gas—lots and lots of gas. Many have found out the hard way that when the juice is stored in a closed container, the quickly decompressed contents can make quite a mess, and the smell stays with you for a long, long, long, long, *long* time. It's a mistake most people make only once.

MILK FEVER

Veterinary medicine doesn't offer many opportunities for instant gratification. Often, after treating an animal, we leave follow-up directions, essentially leaving any ongoing treatment to the farmer. It may be weeks before we learn the fate of one of our patients.

Such is not the case with *parturient paresis*, or *milk fever*. Contrary to what the name implies, the cow's body temperature usually drops a little when suffering from this condition, which means it has about as much to do with fever as John Travolta in a white suit.

But it does have to do with milk. Around the time of calving, blood calcium, and sometimes phosphorus and magnesium too, can get dangerously low. Calcium, besides being the element that gives strength to bones, is an essential component in muscle contraction. Most species experience muscle rigidity when blood calcium falls, but cows are too obstinate for that. They just become weak.

Milk fever happens almost exclusively in dairy cows, with rare exceptions in heavy-milking beef breeds. It also happens almost exclusively within a few days of delivering a calf. When a dairy cow has a calf, she begins to produce milk. In fact, she makes enough milk to feed about four calves. Since milk is rich in calcium and phosphorus, she draws calcium from her bloodstream to put into the milk. She draws it so fast that she may not compensate rapidly enough and her blood calcium falls below a critical level. Once that threshold is reached, she becomes so weak that she can't even stand. It can happen within minutes.

But treating these cows *does* reward the clinician with the unusual prize of instant gratification. It's a dramatic recovery and the treatment is—you guessed it—*calcium*.

As simple as that is, administering the calcium can be a real trick. To get the best results, it has to be introduced directly into the bloodstream. Intravenous calcium injections can cause the heart to do strange things—like stop. The best way to stay on top of the situation is to hook the patient up to a cardiac monitor and keep an eye on things during treatment. If you have any medical training and you know what "hooking up" to a cardiac monitor entails, you might wonder how it's done with cows. It isn't. In fact, I shudder to think what the EKG of a cow receiving an intravenous infusion of calcium would look like. It might scare the cow to death. Rather, we sort of fly by the seat of our pants. It's more art than science, but it does help to run it in slow.

Well, I guess we don't fly *entirely* by the seat of our pants. I do like to keep tabs on the heart rate by monitoring her pulse. Unfortunately, though, if a cow develops complications due to the calcium, her pulse rate will give me about a three-second warning before cardiac arrest occurs. Three seconds isn't a lot of time for remedial action. Fortunately, it's usually a smooth procedure.

After treatment, we usually enjoy the instant gratification of watching the cow stand up after a little mild encouragement. If blood phosphorus is also low, gratification may be delayed by a couple of hours. Still, as medicine goes, that's pretty good.

WOODEN TONGUES AND WEEPY EYES

Heavy-milking beef cows may lose several hundred pounds while raising a calf because of the energy demands of lactation. Once the calf is weaned, however, the good beef cow will gain all that weight back again so she can support another calf the following year. So you can imagine why, when a cow weaned a nice calf but never gained her weight back again, the farmer called me to have a closer look at her.

When I arrived I observed her at the feed bunk. She couldn't quite get the grain in her mouth. She had better luck with hay, but it was a struggle for her to chew it. Then I noticed a few other things. She looked strange. Her coat was sloppy looking, her mouth was a little swollen, and there was debris in her nose. If you've spent some quality time with cattle you know that they're fastidious about their noses. They constantly clean out their nostrils with their tongues. It's gross, sure, but they have very clean nostrils.

There was something else strange about this cow: She kept her mouth closed unless she was trying to eat. I quickly came up with a short list of conditions that I wanted to check during my exam, like *listeriosis* (a bacterial infection), *wooden tongue* (also a bacterial infection), or a broken jaw. Once the halter was on, keeping her under control, I had a look inside her mouth. What I found was quite unexpected.

In medical circles, a rare disease that mimics a common disease is often referred to as a *zebra*. When I was in veterinary school, the wise clinicians told us that if you hear hoof beats, it's probably a horse, not a zebra. In other words, if the signs an animal displays are consistent with common diseases, think of the common ones first.

When I opened the cow's mouth, a zebra reared up and whacked me upside the head. This cow was missing the front third of her tongue. The lack of this important appendage completely prevented her from grazing, as the cow uses her tongue to reach out and grab her bite of grass. It also prevented the patient from eating grain, since the tongue is used to rake the grain into her mouth. She couldn't groom her coat, nor could she keep her nostrils clean. The result makes perfect sense to me now—a cow with a rough hair coat, a dirty nose, and not gaining weight.

I spent some time with the farmer trying to figure out how this could have happened, and the honest truth is that neither one of us had a clue. It wasn't a recent wound as it had completely healed. Maybe aliens beamed down and snatched it for study; I don't know. But lucky for the cow and the farmer, she eventually found a way to compensate and remained in the herd for several more years. As for the hoof beats, this was most definitely a zebra. I saw the stripes with my own eyes.

Then there's the dreaded wooden tongue. I had seen missing tongue, lacerated tongue, and ulcerated tongue, but it was eighteen years before I finally saw wooden tongue. This condition, caused by a bacteria called *Actinobacillus lignieresii,* causes a cow's tongue to swell and take on the consistency of wood. Fortunately, treatment is simple. We gave the drooling heifer a long course of antibiotics and she recovered nicely.

That same day on the same farm, as an afterthought, I was asked to have a look at a heifer with a weepy eye. I've seen hundreds of heifers with weepy eyes and they nearly all have the same type of corneal lesion that responds to a shot of antibiotic. This one, however, didn't have the characteristic cloudiness that we usually see in the cornea. So we caught her up with a halter and, once restrained, I took a good look under her eyelids and found the granddaddy of all grass awns.

One of my professors said, *The grass awn is perhaps one of the most dangerous articles in nature to livestock,* and that pretty much sums it up. A grass awn is a tiny dried seed that usually contains some sort of barb. Nature designed it to latch onto an animal for transport to a distant location. Eventually, it falls off and hits the ground, hoping to germinate in the spring. The grass awn embedded under this cow's eyelid would have dropped my professor in his tracks. If we hadn't caught it in time, it surely would have migrated through her brain on its way to her heart before finally killing her. Grass awns cannot be treated with magnets, so I pulled this one out with a hemostat (a fancy medical name for a pair of tweezers that's specifically designed to compress a blood vessel) and considered getting it mounted by a taxidermist.

WANNA SEE SOMETHING *REALLY* GROSS?

That's a trick question. I have an irrational fear of spiders. I work with big, powerful animals, but those nasty little eight-legged killers freak me out. One morning, I was scanning a group of cows for pregnancy and a spider began its slow descent off of my ultrasound goggles right in front of my face. My ultrasound machine is portable and the picture is viewed through a set of quasi-virtual monitor goggles preventing my view of basically anything else besides the ultrasound picture. But I could see the spider as it dangled for a second—until I tried to blow it away. I gave a couple of panicked breaths until momentum brought the swinging arachnid right back onto the side of my face.

Scanning cows is a dirty job, and the hand not inside of the cow's rear end inevitably gets covered with manure after only a few examinations. One of my hands was still inside the cow and the other one was just as dirty, but I had to make a split-second decision—ignore the spider or wipe it off with my manure-covered glove. Before you could say "yuk," I had a green streak across my face and I was intensely relieved that the spider was gone.

So when I went out to look at a case of *teat spiders* for the first time, you can imagine my trepidation. I really don't know why they're called that because they don't resemble spiders at all. They aren't even alive. They're still kind of gross, but not as gross as real spiders.

Upon examination, I discovered that *teat spider,* or *milk stone,* is a farmer term for a pea-sized concretion inside the cow's teat canal. It has the consistency of wax and is mostly made of calcium and sloughed mammary-gland cells. Whenever this farmer tried to milk his cow, the milk stone would act like a ball valve and occlude the inside of the teat, preventing the flow of milk. It was like a big, fleshy ballpoint pen.

Reestablishing flow in these girls is a bit tricky, and it's really no fun for the cow. The surgeon has to dilate the teat opening slightly with an instrument and try to squeeze the milk stone through the opening. Most of the time this can be accomplished without complication, but sometimes drastic measures have to be taken.

I have seen a couple of these milk stones that were bigger than my little finger. Obviously, passing one this size through the tiny teat orifice is impossible. When that happens I reach for my knife. With a generous amount of local anesthetic, I can make a careful incision along the length of the teat just big enough to fetch the obstructing milk stone. But I have to keep my head on a swivel to avoid flying hooves. The cow doesn't understand the gravity of the situation and just wants me to stop.

MORE BLOCKAGES

Teat canals aren't the only things that can get blocked. The poor cow with a case of the bloat most certainly feels the logjam. Bloat happens when a cow can't burp—and cows burp a *lot*. Their complex digestion through fermentation produces a lot of gas, upwards of a liter or two per minute, and gas production doesn't stop even during an outflow obstruction.

Any number of things can cause bloat. Occasionally, an apple or potato gets stuck in the throat; sometimes the gas simply accumulates within froth similar to suds on a beer. Cows can't burp froth. And sometimes, we don't know why they bloat. Correction involves passing a large bloat tube about the size of a garden hose down the cow's throat. Once in the gas pocket, the block is bypassed and the gas can flow again.

There is an entire field, *bovine obstetrics*, that deals with blockages of the womb. From overly large calves to abnormal presentations, the cow that has difficulty delivering her calf no doubt feels the pressure. One of the most common blockages of the womb is *uterine torsion*, or twisted uterus. As the name implies, the cow's womb literally twists shut, preventing passage of the calf. Uterine torsion is very common in dairy cows because of their anatomy: The deep body and large complex stomach allow the womb to rotate inside the abdomen and get itself trapped in the wrong spot. These unfortunate cows are generally pretty uncomfortable at best and, if the twist is tight enough, in grave danger of death at worst.

Regardless of the severity, a twisted uterus always requires intervention.

LET'S DO THE (UN)TWIST

Cattle farmers, beef and dairy alike, are keenly aware of when their cattle are about to give birth. They must be attentive and prepared, ready to render assistance to any cow that is laboring without progress. As such, the veterinarian is called to fix some accidents of birth that the farmer can't handle on his own.

Uterine torsion, one of the most common complications, is relatively easy for the farmer to recognize, but difficult for him to fix. Here's what it's all about: Imagine a pillowcase as the womb and birth canal. Now shove a pillow into the pillowcase. This represents the calf. Twist the opening of the pillowcase closed by rotating it 180 degrees. Finally, try to remove the pillow through the twisted opening. I bet you can't do it. Neither can the cow.

I go over the four degrees of difficulty of uterine torsion in my mind from the comfort of my truck as I drive out to the farm. The easiest (first degree) is when the vet reaches up into the birth canal and simply flips the calf around. When this happens, I have to stand there and look busy with my gloved arm shoulder-deep in the cow.

I might let out an occasional grunt or make a painful face. After all, I don't want to make it look *too* easy. But the honest truth is that the first-degree twisted uterus is so rare that I have yet to see one. At least that's my story. They do, however, almost always result in a live calf. At least that's what I've been told. I wish we could plan them all that way.

The next most difficult (second degree) twisted uterus is the most common. This is when the uterus is twisted up, but the vet can still get a hand on the calf inside the womb. These take considerable effort to untwist. In fact, I was in practice for five years before I could unwrap one of these without the help of a tool.

To fix these manually, I have to reach into the birth canal and find the calf's head. Once that's done I summon all of my upper body strength and rock the calf in the opposite direction of the twist. After about twenty or thirty seconds of this I usually take a break. It's a major effort and I can only keep it up for so long. Then I reach in with my other arm and try again. Then I stop, take a quick break, and try again with the original arm. If several rounds of this produce no results it's time to resort to plan B.

If there's enough help on the farm, like three or four young, fearless scrappy farmhands, we can cast the cow on the ground and roll her over. We roll her in the same direction as the twist while placing a knee over where the calf is in her belly. It seems counterintuitive, but we really do roll her in the same direction as the twist. I think of it as rolling the cow around the twisted calf. We just have to make sure we definitively know the direction of the twist or things could get *really* complicated.

And if we don't have adequate manpower or horsepower to roll the cow over (it's not an easy job), we can always reach for the de-torsion rod. This appropriately named instrument looks like something out of an enhanced interrogator's toolbox. It's a two-foot-long steel bar with an eye loop at each end. My professors in veterinary school discouraged its use. They said the only thing it was good for was chasing away the dogs that harass us while we're trying to untwist a uterus. There's a good reason: It has earned a bad reputation for breaking the legs of the calf. If you're going to use it you have to be very careful and you have to know what you're doing.

To use it, the practitioner places an obstetrical chain around each of the calf's front feet, or it's rear if it's backwards. He crisscrosses them through the first loop of the rod and again through the second loop. Once pulled tight, a screwdriver or similar tool is placed in the outside eye of the rod for leverage and, with a steady rotation, the calf and the uterus are unrolled.

Regardless if the twist was corrected manually, by rolling the cow with the bare (okay, *gloved*) hands, or with the help of a rod, the second-degree torsion always ends with a natural delivery of the calf through the birth canal. One can always be guaranteed of a slimy, wet, stinky shirt sleeve and a painful, sore shoulder in need of an ice pack after correcting one of these. Unfortunately, a live calf is never a guarantee with a second-degree twist, despite the best planning.

I always hope for a second-degree torsion whenever I'm called to fix a twisted uterus. The next two are quite difficult and the first-degree twist doesn't exist, at least not that I'll admit. But hope is never a strategy for obstetrical corrections, so I have to be prepared for the colossal difficulties of the third degree twisted uterus, the one where a natural delivery through the birth canal is not possible without endangering the life of the cow. When I determine that there is no chance of untwisting the uterus by any accepted method, or maybe because there is no evidence that the cow will dilate normally, the only safe option is surgery. Meet the third degree.

A barn is not an ideal operating theater, and a cesarean section is fraught with danger for the cow. The procedure is time-consuming, so every second that her insides are exposed to the outside increases the likelihood of her insides becoming infected, and an infected inside never ends well for the cow. Also, the hole we cut into her side has to be large enough for a hundred-pound calf to fit through, fourteen inches minimum. In other words, it's a little more extreme than a human C-section. A fourteen-inch incision has more opportunity to break down before it's completely healed, and that never ends well for the cow either.

The fourth-degree uterine torsion is the worst kind. These are the ones that can't be fixed at all except with the type of heroic means that become cost-prohibitive. Some cows may have a uterus that rolls beyond 360 degrees. When it gets this tight, blood supply to the uterus becomes compromised, the tissue dies and the pain may temporarily stop for the patient. In the short term, she might not even show any sign that there's a problem, but within a couple of days she begins to develop toxins in her bloodstream which, naturally, make her sick. When this happens we have little choice but to euthanize the cow.

So I wonder, as I drive to the farm for a twisted uterus call, which degree it will be. One evening, when I arrived on the farm, my patient, number 99, was haltered to a post. The farmer said that he hoped for an easy one and I enthusiastically agreed. As I reached in, I was still going over the possibilities in my head. *Please don't let this be a C-section!*

Fortunately, the first thing I felt was the head of the calf. The patient's water hadn't broken yet. This was good news as it indicated that a natural delivery through the birth canal was likely. I popped through the amniotic membrane and relieved the patient of a few gallons of slippery fetal fluids, thereby making a mess and, coincidentally, lightening the load for manual correction.

After draining as much of the fluid as I could, I put my arm on top of the calf's head and started to push down in a counterclockwise direction. I began to rock it around and, sure enough, I got tired before I could make any progress. I abandoned all hope that this would be an easy first-degree twisted uterus (as if they even exist). I thought maybe my other arm could do better, so I donned another shoulder-length glove and reached in.

Once again, I worked until fatigue set in. My plan was falling apart. It's usually about this time that I start to consider that I might have to roll the cow, or even break out the de-torsion rod taboo. Then the inevitable thoughts raced through my head about having to resort to a C-section. Nobody likes a C-section, but would this one be necessary? Then, on my third try, *boom*. The calf flipped.

The only guarantees with a second-degree twisted uterus are a slimy, stinky shirt sleeve and a tired, sore shoulder. A live birth is never guaranteed. So we still had work to do. I attached the obstetrical chains and delivered a big, slimy heifer with the assistance of the farmer and a rope. Once on the ground, the calf took the first breath of life.

I love it when a plan comes together.

ENDING ON A HIGH NOTE

Before a cow can give birth it first must be *with calf*. Today's farms are filled with newfangled technologies that yesterday's farmers never could have imagined. In fact, far from the backward image that many Americans have, modern farmers are high-tech early adopters, embracing new ways of doing things and applying them to every aspect of agriculture and animal husbandry, to include breeding. Yes, I'm saying that bovine romance literally isn't what it used to be. Artificial insemination of cattle is the new standard and it is responsible for much of the genetic improvement of livestock realized over the last several decades. Nowadays, many farmers even utilize *embryo transfer* and *in vitro fertilization* to exploit the superior traits of some of their top females in the herd. The process can get rather expensive, and there are no guarantees that the end result—multiple live calves in a short amount of time from a single female—may be accomplished, but here's how it's supposed to work.

The eggs are collected from the cow's ovaries and prepared in a lab to be fertilized. Once fertilized with sperm selected to produce only female calves, the resulting embryos are cultured in an incubator for one week until they are mature enough to be transferred into recipient animals. The recipient animals become pregnant, carry the calves to term, and deliver the new calves into the world. It sounds simple, but it's incredibly complicated and expensive.

A client of mine recently embarked on this adventure. The process is technically challenging, and there is no room for error during any of the numerous steps in the process, so when we collected from several donor cows and multiple pregnancies resulted, everyone was ecstatic. Well, at least the people were; I'm making an assumption about the cows. They don't talk.

As the old adage goes, however, don't count your chickens before they hatch. Or, more appropriately, don't count your calves before the recipients deliver them. One of the donors produced three pregnant recipients which usually would mean three live heifer calves since the sperm used to fertilize the eggs had been selected to produce only females. During the routine ultrasound of the pregnancies, we discovered that one of the pregnancies was actually a bull. Surprise! In reality, it's about ninety percent effective.

Okay, chalk that one up to bad luck; two out of three still isn't too bad. Unfortunately, six months later, another one of the recipients went into labor early and lost the other pregnancy. There's still one left. We crossed our fingers.

Finally, the farmer called me early one morning to help deliver the last remaining calf. The cow was in labor, but couldn't deliver on her own. At the same time, I was informed that the embryo donor had died the previous month in a freak barn accident, so this was our last chance to get a live heifer calf from her. No pressure.

I arrived at the farm and did the normal examination. The calf's head was twisted backwards preventing her from entering the birth canal. I was able to correct the position of the calf, but it seemed awfully big and the mama cow was, well, *not* very big.

It took us about two seconds to decide that, in this case, a C-section was the only viable option. We walked her in the barn and delivered the calf, alive and well, through the cow's side. When all was said and done, the farmer and I took a seat and watched the calf take her first wobbly steps while her mother licked her clean. It was a good day for everyone, even if I did get poop on my shoes.

CONCLUSION

When it comes to the types of meat that we favor,
chicken takes the number-one spot, but beef takes pride
of place. Fried chicken is good, but no one makes chicken
steaks, restaurants do not tempt us with sizzling platters
of inch-thick cuts of poultry, and we don't obsess over the
exquisite marbling of the humble chicken wing. For the
most part, we save that kind of care, attention, and even
admiration, for beef and beef alone.

In the ancient world, and even among some
societies in the 21st century, it was believed that consuming
meat imparted the qualities possessed by the donor animal.
Eating a cheetah or a gazelle granted speed, eating a
kangaroo made you jumpy, eating a lion conferred nobility
and ferocity, and eating a sloth made you, well, *slothful*.
(No word on which qualities the chicken would impart.)

All of this gives me pause. Maybe the benefits of
eating beef aren't purely nutritional and flavorful. Maybe
beef helps make us who we are on a higher level. Think

about it: Cows are curious. Curiosity drives human achievement. Cows are stoic. Humans have endured untold millennia of hardship and challenge. Cows care for their young with vigor and intensity, just like human mothers. Cows can be irritable and demanding of their personal space, just like people. Cows are allelomimetic. (Remember that one? I should have warned you there'd be a test.) Humans engage in more mimicry than we'd like to admit; in fact, the ability to quickly learn behaviors and habits from one another is a key to our success. But if we inherit all of these behaviors from our bovine cousins, one trait that we surely don't share is intelligence. Or maybe we do and we've been kidding ourselves all this time.

I am not a particularly profound person, nor do I think I am particularly wise, but I do have an inclination to view the world through a lens to a barnyard. So, if I could offer a tidbit of advice, my advice would be to . . . wait for it . . . be like a cow.

Did you expect anything different after reading this book? But, admittedly, my advice sounds less like wisdom and more like folly. How is it good advice to be like a cow? I mean, cows are large, high-strung, lumbering vegetarians. Urging someone to be like a cow doesn't exactly resemble sound advice.

But since I look through the lens of a window to a barnyard, there are attributes of cows from which we can garner wisdom, but only if we pay attention to their peculiarities.

Cows are curious animals, and a natural curiosity is essential for anyone interested in ongoing personal development. Satisfying a curiosity about the way things are is how a cow learns, and learning is essential. Cows investigate any and all things to which they have access, like the feed bunk, the person standing in the scrape alley, or the porcupine that just wandered into the pasture. The electric fence is also an object of curiosity, so be careful of the things you try.

Cows are hard-working critters and I don't think anyone would dispute that. The beef cow with a calf at her side works hard to feed, protect, and raise that calf until it's old enough to be set on its own. Pound for pound, the dairy cow expends as many calories to produce the milk she gives as a runner does to run a marathon; she does this every day. She's a real worker and the farmer appreciates her effort. But if a dairy cow gets lazy and doesn't make milk, she will likely lose her job.

Cows also like to rest. That is not antithetical to being a hard worker; it is necessary. If a cow doesn't take a rest by lying down and chewing on the cud for a spell, she won't get all she can out of her feed. It is through her feed, after all, that she makes her living by converting forage to protein. Too much time on her feet can lead to hoof trouble. Lying down allows for proper circulation. A good rest, in moderation, will leave the cow ready to capitalize fully on her opportunities.

Speaking of a good rest, cows are entitled to a vacation once in a while. The dairy cow, when she is pregnant and her milk production is decreasing rapidly, gets a lactation vacation that lasts a month or two. That might seem excessive to a person like you or me, but it is necessary for the cow to regenerate her mammary tissue. It's done in anticipation of her next lactation and, without it, she just won't be very productive.

But there is a limit. Vacations that last more than a couple of months can result in a cow that becomes soft and squishy. That's not exactly the right condition to prepare for the metabolic marathons she is about to run.

Cows are social critters, and so are we. They stick together during mealtime, during rest time, and when it's time to move to greener pastures. In fact, one way we can tell a cow just isn't herself is when she lags behind the rest of the herd. This bovine social interaction is cow-to-cow, not virtual. So, while social media may have a place, it isn't a substitute for a face-to-face meeting, a firm handshake, or an in-person visit to a friend.

Indeed, cows are social animals and they create a necessary social order within every herd. Whenever the order is disturbed, like when a new group of animals is introduced, the order must be reestablished. There are no exceptions to this. Cows always pick a leader; she's known as the boss cow.

But there is only one leader, and power struggles are common until the leader is established. Not every cow can be the boss. Once the conflicts have been worked out, and they eventually *do* get worked out, the herd lives with a relative lack of conflict.

Lack of conflict is not equivalent to peace, though. We all have to pick leaders at work, associations, clubs, or government. Once the boss cow is picked, the herd is pretty much stuck with her. The only term limit available is when another cow dethrones her. So, pick your leaders with careful and honest consideration.

Cows are nurturing mothers; well, the good ones are anyway. Nurturing ability doesn't have to be exclusive to moms, though; there are other things to nurture besides offspring. Continuing education needs nurturing, just like with your career, your health, and your relationships with your fellow man and your God.

Can cows be a model for good human development, something to which we should aspire? Even I'll admit that's taking it a bit too far, and I really dig cows. We have to look past some things like the constant drooling and belching, the inclination to fear the unknown, and tendency to deposit manure wherever and whenever. But if you dig deep enough, you'll find some useful nuggets of cow wisdom.

Here's one more: As Thomas de Quincey said, *Cows are amongst the gentlest of breathing creatures,* which I guess means that Mr. de Quincey was excluding plants. But, defensive actions aside (and who can blame them for that?), he was right. Cows are gentle, amiable, and peaceful, unless they are in the working chute. My teenage daughter would say they are *chill*. They share the barnyard and, for the most part, they get along with one another. They even get along with us. Maybe this is the one bovine trait where the cows are ahead of the curve.

These are the things I think about when I'm trudging through ankle-deep manure, fixing a prolapsed uterus, delivering a stubborn calf, treating an infected wound, or wandering around a rainy barnyard with a worried farmer. I'm one of the links that holds the entire network of food, farmers, and families together. Veterinarians and veterinary science have been, and continue to be, major contributors to the increasingly productive American farm. We are partners with the people and the animals who provide a secure food supply for over three hundred and twenty-eight million people seven days a week. The families, the farms, the animals, and the medicine are inseparable from one another. It's humbling to be a link in that chain, but I'm proud to be a part of it. I wouldn't do anything else. So thanks for spending some time with me, the farmers, and the cows. We enjoyed the company, and we appreciate your interest in learning a little more about a world that most Americans know very little about, yet literally sustains all of our lives. Maybe it changed your perspective a little, or maybe you learned a few new things that you can bring up at dinner tomorrow. Or maybe it inspired you to consider a new career. I sure hope so. And I hope that the next time you bite into a delicious hamburger or carve into a juicy steak, you raise a glass of ice-cold milk to a farmer because, when it comes right down to it, your food was grown somewhere by a farmer.

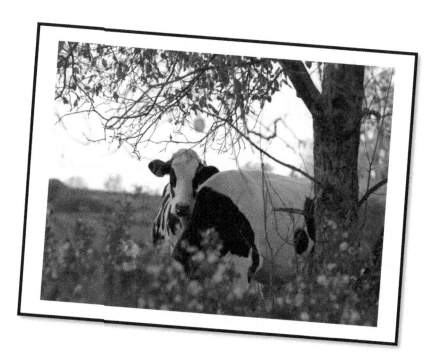

ACKNOWLEDGEMENTS

Writing the acknowledgements for a book, at least a book written by me, is a daunting task. It's not because I have no one to thank; on the contrary, I have a lot of people to thank.

My wife, life partner, soul mate, and best friend, Sheila, with her quiet patience and understanding has allowed me to pursue professional opportunities with the fullest of passion in order to serve our clients, the farmers. She has not only tolerated my profession but embraced it. Our children, Nolan and Bena, have endured my occasional absence from the soccer games, dance recitals, and the dinner table for most their lives. I suspect it may be the reason neither of them desires to follow in my footsteps.

My parents, Bill and Liz Croushore, laid the foundation for the success of my brother and me through their patience, love, and sacrifice. Their devotion to family is something to behold.

In the fall of 2009, the Somerset, Pennsylvania *Daily American* agreed to print my weekly column. I was warned that maintaining a weekly column would be a challenge, and the warnings were true; it has been a challenge. But the column was well received, and I am extremely grateful to the *Daily American*, its editor Brian Whipkey, and my main contact for ten years, Brian Schrock, for their encouragement and support. I am also heartened by and grateful for the readers who have likened me to writers with whom I have no business being compared. This book is drawn from the articles that have appeared over the years in that column, "The View from the Back 40."

I am blessed to have had many smart, practical, and hard-working mentors in my veterinary career and trying to acknowledge them all by name would be an exercise in futility. If one spends any amount of time reflecting on the influence others have had upon our lives, it becomes glaringly obvious that our individual achievements are possible only because of the influence, and often the sacrifice, of others. My entire skill set is built upon that which existed well before I began my veterinary education. But the individual mentorship of experienced colleagues has been so essential to any measure of the success I have achieved that I credit them entirely with who I have become as a clinician. I will not attempt to name any of my mentors individually, but suffice it to say that I have learned something from the first veterinarian whom I visited while exploring the profession as a career choice, to the most recent colleague I consulted for help on a difficult case. The people of this profession are so diverse and dynamic that my zeal for veterinary medicine grows with every new encounter.

While at a book signing in the fall of 2019, I had a serendipitous encounter with someone who introduced me to Jason Liller. Without the help and guidance of Jason, this book, literally, would not have been possible. He has the uncanny ability to assemble the pieces of a puzzle that, at first glance, don't look like they should fit together. Yet, once arranged, they form a picture that that should have been obvious, like being shown the answer to a brain teaser after getting stuck trying to solve it.

Pastoral images of farm settings are comforting to many of us but capturing their reality and beauty at the same time is not easy. There are few people whom I know that make it look easy and the some of the pictures seen in this book were taken by her. Jess VanGilder is not a professional photographer, but if the whole farming thing doesn't work out, she sure could be. I thank her for her contribution to this book.

My partner at our veterinary practice, Dr. Dan Zawisza, has taken the heat off me so I can pursue often hare-brained ideas, like advanced reproductive technologies in domestic livestock, and writing books. Our former partner and practice founder, Dr. David Welch, offered me a position with the practice almost two decades ago and set before me a deep well from which to draw good water. For both, I am extremely grateful.

Pastoral images of farm settings are comforting to many of us but capturing their reality and beauty at the same time is not easy. There are few people whom I know that make it look easy and the pictures on the cover were taken by her. Jess VanGilder is not a professional photographer, but if the whole farming thing doesn't work out, she sure could be. I thank her for the contribution for the cover of this book.

In the last several years, the scope of my practice has evolved to include significant travel to farms across the region where we perform various embryo-transfer techniques employed by farmers who wish to improve their herds. This sort of work requires friendly, reliable, and skilled assistants whom I employ and travel with. Jenny Coleman and Ashley Kaufman both fit this bill and, without their help and willingness to take their turns behind the wheel so I can tickle the keys of the laptop, I would have never even attempted this book.

Finally, the American farmers, with their skill, persistence, work ethic, and dedication to their way of life, provide the raw material for life-sustaining nourishment for the rest of us. Often misunderstood and underestimated, they do the work on which we all depend, the work that allows the rest of us to eat. Farmers have achieved a high level of sophistication that rivals any other endeavor, yet are often perceived as naive and uneducated. I have learned more from farmers about life than I could ever teach them about veterinary medicine.

ABOUT DR. CROUSHORE

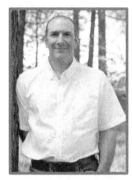 **Dr. Bill Croushore** was raised in Ruffsdale, Westmoreland County, in southwestern Pennsylvania. He graduated from Duquesne University School of Pharmacy in 1992 and practiced pharmacy in southwestern Virginia until 1993 when he enrolled in the Virginia-Maryland Regional College of Veterinary Medicine (Virginia Tech), receiving his doctorate in 1997.

Dr. Croushore's professional interests include embryo transfer, pushing the limits of on farm oocyte collection (cow eggs), herd health management and bovine surgery. He has been certified by the American Embryo Transfer Association for exporting bovine embryos internationally since 2012 and he holds membership in the American Veterinary Medical Association, Pennsylvania Veterinary Medical Association, American Association of Bovine Practitioners, the Society for Theriogenology,

American Embryo Transfer Association, and the International Embryo Transfer Society. He is a member of the board of directors of the American Embryo Transfer Association and served the association as secretary-treasurer in 2019. He is also the treasurer for the Somerset County Holstein Association and is a member of the Berlin Brothersvalley School District Ag Advisory Committee.

Dr. Croushore writes a weekly column in the *Somerset Daily American* entitled "The View from the Back 40." He is also a regular contributor to *Pinzgauer Journal* and the *Keystone Cattleman.* His first published book, *Oops, . . . And Other Words You Don't Like to Hear Your Surgeon Say,* was released in the summer of 2018.

When not engaged in professional activities, he enjoys time with his family, hunting the often-elusive whitetail deer, and fishing. Dr. Croushore is married to Sheila, his wife of twenty-five years, and is the proud father of two children, Nolan (nineteen) and Bena (fifteen). He attends St. Peter's Roman Catholic Church where he teaches eighth-grade CCD.

ABOUT JASON LILLER

After serving in the US Air Force during the First Gulf War, Jason Liller made the fateful decision to visit his local bookstore and ask for a job, beginning a thirty-year odyssey of bookselling, publishing, writing, and editing.

Recruited by the legendary Charlie "Tremendous" Jones, Jason spent almost twenty years helping run his publishing company. Today, Jason continues his mission to help people get their ideas into print, working with New York Times bestselling authors like Ken Blanchard, Bob Burg, Mark Sanborn, and Jim Stovall, and he's turned first-draft manuscripts into fully realized books that have sold hundreds of thousands of copies.

Jason lives with his family in Mechanicsburg, Pennsylvania in a home stockpiled with caffeine, dog treats, and zillions of books.

GET BACK TO THE BARNYARD WITH DR. BILL!

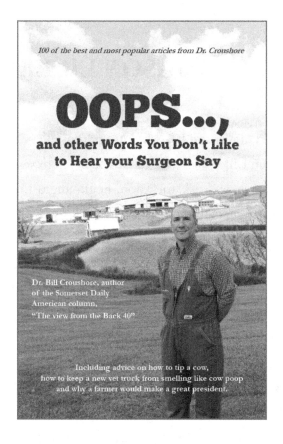

100 of the best and most popular articles from Dr. Croushore

OOPS...,
and other Words You Don't Like to Hear your Surgeon Say

Dr. Bill Croushore, author of the Somerset Daily American column, "The view from the Back 40"

Including advice on how to tip a cow, how to keep a new vet truck from smelling like cow poop and why a farmer would make a great president.

Learn the finer points of cow tipping, how to keep your new truck from smelling like cow poop, and why a farmer would make a great president in Dr. Bill Croushore's first book, *Oops . . ., and Other Words You Don't Like to Hear Your Surgeon Say,* a collection of his popular *Somerset Daily American* column "The View from the Back 40."

**AVAILABLE NOW from
www.MadeInSomersetCounty.com and
www.Amazon.com**

Made in the USA
Middletown, DE
22 May 2021

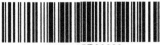